DYNAMIC LIVING

Formerly entitled *Lifestyle Capsules*

Aileen Ludington, MD
Hans Diehl, DrHSc, MPH

Lifestyle Medicine Institute
Loma Linda, California

REVIEW AND HERALD® PUBLISHING ASSOCIATION
HAGERSTOWN, MD 21740

Edited by Darryl Ludington and Raymond H. Woolsey
Interior design by Richard Tinker
Cover design by Mark Bond
Cover photo by The Stock Market/Chuck Savage
Sectional Illustrations by Elyse Whittaker
Typeset in 11/15 Helvetica Light

Published and distributed by
Review and Herald® Publishing Association

Distributed simultaneously in Canada.
Printed in the United States of America.

Library of Congress Cataloging in Publication Data

Ludington, Aileen.
    Dynamic Living : the best current health knowledge in 52 concise information pack-
ets / Aileen Ludington, Hans Diehl.
    p. cm.
    Includes index.
    1. Health.   2. Medicine, Popular.   I. Diehl, Hans, 1946-
II. Title.
RA776.L9595 1993
613—dc20
                                                                            91-9139
                                                                            CIP

99   98   97   96   95   5   4   3   2

ISBN 0-8280-0949-X

A Significant Impact

"*Dynamic Living* is a feature that has had a significant impact on readers of award-winning *Signs of the Times* magazine. All the 'capsules' that appeared in *Signs* are in this book—and many more besides."
—*Kenneth J. Holland, former editor,* Signs of the Times.

Clarity, Charm, and Thoroughness

"The greatest challenge of Western medicine is to educate and motivate patients to adopt a healthier lifestyle. *Dynamic Living* is doing exactly that—with clarity, charm, and thoroughness."
—*William Castelli, MD, director, Framingham Heart Study.*

Extend Your Life

"These are important concepts that, when internalized, will do more to improve your health and extend your life than all the technological wonders of modern medicine."
—*John McDougall, MD, internist and author,*
McDougall's Medicine *and other best-sellers.*

On the Cutting Edge

"The authors are totally reliable and on the cutting edge of lifestyle medicine."
—*Denis Burkitt, MD, London.*

No One Can Read and Remain the Same

"The authors have been in the forefront of preventive medicine since long before it was fashionable. They confront health questions and anxieties with compelling evidence and grace. No one can read even a few of these chapters and remain the same."
—*Herbert E. Douglass, ThD, former president, Weimar Institute.*

A Solid Book

"Solid book, clearly written, providing a sensible introduction to the basis of natural health management."
—*John Robbins, author,* Diet for a New America.

The Most Practical Key

"This may be the most practical key to a better lifestyle that many of us have ever found."
—*Dan Matthews, executive producer/host,* Lifestyle Magazine.

Hans Diehl, DrHSc, MPH

As a National Institutes of Health-sponsored research fellow in cardiovascular epidemiology at Loma Linda University, Dr. Diehl evaluated the impact of the Pritikin Longevity Center, where he served as director of the Research and Health Education program.

As a post-doctoral scholar at the School of Public Health at the University of California at Los Angeles, he contributed to the establishment of the UCLA Center for Health Enhancement. He holds a doctorate in Health Science with emphasis on lifestyle medicine and has a master's degree in Public Health Nutrition from Loma Linda University.

Dr. Diehl is the founder and director of the Lifestyle Medicine Institute in Loma Linda, California. He is editor of *Lifeline Health Letter,* health columnist for several publications, and author of the bestseller *To Your Health.* He has demonstrated and published results showing that many hypertensives, diabetics and heart disease patients can normalize their disease and become drug-free within weeks by simplifying their customary rich Western diet.

Dr. Diehl travels widely as a seminar leader and appears frequently on TV and radio.

Aileen Ludington, MD

Dr. Ludington, a graduate of Loma Linda University, is a board-certified physician with 25 years of practice experience. Her lifelong interest in health education eventually led to a staff appointment at Weimar Institute's residential NEWSTART® Lifestyle Center. There she observed and documented the remarkable clinical improvements in patients with circulatory and degenerative diseases in response to healthful lifestyle changes.

Dr. Ludington spent seven years as medical advisor for the *Westbrook Hospital* television series. She is presently a health columnist for several publications, associate editor of *Lifeline Health Letter,* and medical director of the Lifestyle Medicine Institute in Loma Linda. Dr. Ludington is a popular radio and seminar speaker, particularly in the area of weight control. She recently completed her third book.

Dedicated . . .

To NEWSTART® Lifestyle Center and other such live-in programs that demonstrate, month by month, with real people, that the principles presented in this book really work.

To the many faithful participants in our own Lifestyle Medicine Institute seminars who continue to validate these principles in their daily lives.

Caution:

The information in this book is not intended to replace medical advice or treatment. Questions about symptoms and medications, general or specific, should be addressed to your physician.

Contents

Weight Control

Understanding Food

Emotional Health

Natural Remedies

Summary

Index   202

*The first letter of these words together form the acrostic NEWSTART. See page 200.

Preface

In today's world, people can do more for their own health than any doctor, hospital, or technological advance. The scientific data confirms that the choices we make, hour by hour, day by day, largely determine the state of our health, the diseases we get, and often even when we will die. The challenge is to educate, motivate, and inspire people to replace health-destructive habits with health-enhancing lifestyles.

The profusion of health information flowing through the media is overwhelming, confusing, and often contradictory. Today's breakthroughs often become tomorrow's big busts. People long for common sense information that is reliable, understandable, and scientifically sound.

Dynamic Living speaks to that need. In this book, a broad range of health information has been broken down into 52 brief, concise chapters. Study one chapter each week and do its corresponding workbook exercise. At the end of a year you will not only look better and feel younger, but you will have a sound, basic knowledge of nutritional principles, the causes and treatments of today's common diseases, and a clear understanding of how to manage your own life for maximum health and well-being.

HEALTH OUTLOOK

- *Balance*
- *Costs*
- *Western Diet*
- *Nutrition*
- *Children*
- *Aging*

Balance

Chapter 1
Too Many Carrots

I t was headline news: Carrots may prevent head and neck cancer. New research suggests that eating five or six of the crunchy tubers a day appears to reverse leukoplakia—a precancerous lesion occurring in the mouth and throat.

My friend Judith promptly purchased a machine that turned fresh carrots into juice.

"How much juice do you get from five carrots?" I asked her one day.

Her eyes flashed. "Oh, I don't stop there. With this machine I can drink five or six pounds of carrots every day!"

Was that a good idea?

It's true that vegetables are an important part of a healthful diet. It's also true that they are increasingly being valued for their role in preventing disease.

But five pounds of one vegetable every day?

Judith's body eventually rebelled. Her skin took on a sickly yellowish color. Fearing hepatitis, she rushed to the doctor. He explained that carrots contain an orange-yellow dye known as beta-carotene. The body handles reasonable quantities of this substance, but excessive amounts are stashed away in the liver, skin, and mucous membranes, turning them the color of a carrot.

Did that experience straighten her out?

For the moment. But we humans are a curious lot. Sensationalized discoveries and quick solutions to complex health problems are almost irresistible. Before the carrot caper, Judith was swept into the excitement over oat bran. After months of mush and muffins, however, she was ready for a change.

Do carrots actually protect us from cancer?

Carrots and other yellow fruits and vegetables are rich in beta-carotene, the substance that began to change Judith's skin color. Beta-carotene, which the body turns into vitamin A, is also a substance that appears to protect the body against certain cancers.

Vitamins can be divided into two basic types—those that are water-soluble (dissolve in water) and those that are fat-soluble (dissolve in fat). Water-soluble vitamins (B-complex and C) are not a special concern, because excess amounts can usually be washed out through the kidneys.

But fat-soluble vitamins (A, D, E and K) are another story. Any excess cannot be eliminated except as it is used. In excessive amounts, vitamin A begins to act like a toxin (poison) and may cause headaches, joint pains, damaged skin and hair loss. Because of this potential toxicity, laws now limit the amount of vitamin A and other fat-soluble vitamins that can be put into supplements.

Beta-carotene apparently doesn't have such limits. When the body receives beta-carotene it can make as much vitamin A as it needs and use the rest in other ways. That's why the trend these days is to substitute beta-carotene for vitamin A in vitamin capsules and tablets.

This distinction is important because it illustrates how the body uses food. Vitamins, minerals, and other nutrients in natural food occur in exactly the right forms for the body to use. It can pick and choose what it needs. But when we consume one food or nutrient in excess, or tamper with the make-up of food, the whole balance can be upset.

So beta-carotene is good, but a whole lot of it isn't necessarily better.

This is a hard message for today's world. People do nearly everything to excess—they eat too much, drink too much, smoke too much, spend too much, party too much. *Moderation* is about as popular a concept as *wholesome.*

Then too, we live in an instant society with a quick-fix mentality, and it's difficult to accept that instant good health isn't also available. Each time a new fad splashes through the media there's no shortage of takers.

When I was a consultant for a popular health publication, I'd get a lot of phone calls from reporters. They'd try to get me to say things such as: "Yes, eating a pound of alfalfa sprouts every day will strengthen the heart," or "Several capsules of rooted seaweed will ensure a good night's sleep." No one wanted to hear my message about the good sense, balanced diet the body really needs. I soon realized that even though I was giving them the right stuff, a healthful, balanced lifestyle didn't grab headlines, sell magazines (even health magazines) or create profitable new markets for food products.

The human body is able to tolerate excesses of one kind or another for a long time—even six pounds of carrots a day! But the bottom line is that balance, not only in what we eat, but in our total lifestyle, is the key to enduring health and happiness.

Chapter 2

The Dollar$ and $ense of Wellness

America's three leading car makers pay more for health insurance than they do for steel—an astonishing average of $1,650 (1994) per car. With health care costs rising faster than any other item in the Consumer Price Index, more and more companies are learning that ailing employees lead to ailing profits.

What makes employees sick?

Outside of on-the-job hazards, the biggest threat to an employee's health can be his own lifestyle. Studies have convincingly demonstrated that a rich diet, sedentary living, drinking, and smoking largely determine the risk for developing heart disease, stroke, diabetes, cirrhosis of the liver, and cancer of the lungs, breast, prostate, and colon. For instance:

- Smokers at Dow Chemical, when compared to nonsmokers, had six days more absenteeism, eight days more disability and 12 percent more illness, costing the company $1,900 to $2,300 more per smoker per year.

- A significant productivity loss occurs in the 30-49 age group, mostly alcohol related.

- 45 million employees suffer from high blood pressure; this costs industry $3 billion a year. The annual price tag for blood pressure medications and clinical management alone averages about $900 per person.

- A heart attack can cost from $40,000 to $100,000 for medical care and wages lost over a four-month period for a non-management employee.

Can lifestyle changes cut health care costs?

Yes! When Dallas schoolteachers enrolled in a fitness program they averaged three fewer sick days per year. This saved the school district half a million dollars just in substitute pay.

Over a 5-year period, to give another example, the Lockheed Missile and Space Company estimates that its wellness program has saved $1 million in life insurance costs alone. During this period, absenteeism decreased 60 percent, hypertension dropped nearly 90 percent, and employee turnover rates have decreased significantly.

Interest in healthier lifestyles is growing. Alcohol, tobacco, and red meat consumption has markedly gone down and continues dropping, along with mortality figures for heart attacks and strokes. Wellness incentives are being written into many health care plans.

How can employees be encouraged to do what's good for them?

Here are some creative ideas already being tried:

- One property management company pays workers $10 per overweight pound lost and kept off for a six-month period, a $500 bonus to those who stop smoking, and $500 to employees who adopt and follow a regular exercise program.

- A nationwide hospital corporation pays participants 24 cents for each mile run or walked, or four miles biked.

- A large lumber company awards two extra hours of pay each

month to a worker who is not ill or late. If fewer than four days have been missed during a year, a $300 bonus is paid.

The stereotypical businessman—overweight, exhausted, living on cigarettes and three-martini lunches—is out of date. In today's business world, *sweat* is status, and *trimness* is success. More and more modern executives are apt to be in prime condition; neither they nor their companies can afford otherwise.

The message is clear: people are a company's most valuable asset, and they are worth the investment it takes to keep them healthy. Healthy workers accomplish more, and they cost the company less. Anything a company can do to encourage the health of its workers makes sound *dollar$* and good *$en$e*.

From Kernel to Colonel

Forty percent of America's food dollars are spent *eating out.* Our food is processed, refined, concentrated, sugared, salted, and chemically engineered to produce high-calorie, low-nutrient taste sensations. Our cattle are fattened in feedlots without exercise and with antibiotics and growth enhancers. The result: bigger cattle producing juicier steaks containing nearly twice the fat as range-fed cattle. And we are paying dearly for these *advancements.* While we eat to live, what we eat is killing us.

Are you saying food can cause disease?

The statistics are pretty convincing. One hundred years ago, around 10-15 percent of Americans died from coronary heart disease and strokes. Today it's around 40 percent. Back then, less than 6 percent died of cancer, while today the figure is approaching 26 percent.

This isn't *nature's way.* We weren't meant to die in such numbers from heart attacks, strokes, diabetes, and colon and breast cancer. Significant cardiovascular disease began to emerge in America after World War I. It became really rampant after World War II when people could afford diets rich in animal products, and when the food

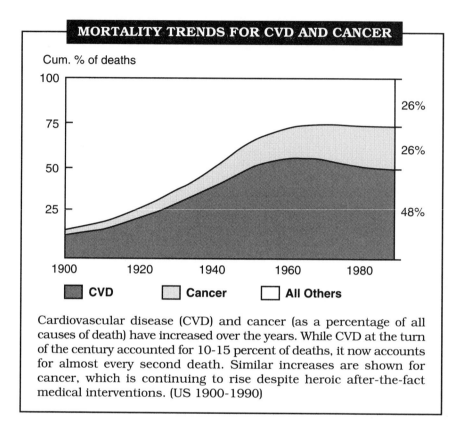

MORTALITY TRENDS FOR CVD AND CANCER

Cum. % of deaths

CVD ◼ Cancer ☐ All Others ☐

Cardiovascular disease (CVD) and cancer (as a percentage of all causes of death) have increased over the years. While CVD at the turn of the century accounted for 10-15 percent of deaths, it now accounts for almost every second death. Similar increases are shown for cancer, which is continuing to rise despite heroic after-the-fact medical interventions. (US 1900-1990)

industry began producing highly processed foods crammed with calories and emptied of nutrition.

Could this be coincidental?

Hardly. This problem is unique to Westernized peoples. Rural populations in China, Japan, and Southeast Asia who have little access to rich foods experience few heart attacks. Similarly, most people in rural Africa and South and Central America have little fear of diabetes and cardiovascular disease. Yet in North America, Australia, New Zealand, and the increasingly affluent countries in Europe and Asia, where diets are rich in fat, heart disease and diabetes are epidemic.

The villains, low fiber and high fat, take their toll by damaging the body's vital oxygen-carrying arteries and by upsetting important metabolic functions. Because of thickened, narrowed arteries, 4,000 Americans have heart attacks every day, every third adult has high blood pressure and thousands are crippled from strokes. Because of disordered metabolisms from unbalanced lifestyles, obesity is epidemic, and a new diabetic is diagnosed every 50 seconds.

How did these dietary changes come about?

Before the turn of the century, the American diet consisted mostly of foods grown in local gardens and nearby farms, supplemented with a few staples from the general store and meat from barnyard animals and range-fed cattle. Our grandparents didn't have thousands of beautifully packaged and highly promoted food products waiting at the supermarket. Fast food restaurants didn't beckon from nearly every street corner.

The backbone of the diet was kernels—kernels of wheat and other grains growing in reassuring profusion. Families ate freshly cooked food and thick slices of home-baked bread around their own

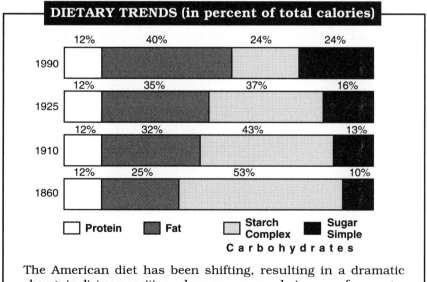

DIETARY TRENDS (in percent of total calories)

	Protein	Fat	Starch Complex	Sugar Simple
1990	12%	40%	24%	24%
1925	12%	35%	37%	16%
1910	12%	32%	43%	13%
1860	12%	25%	53%	10%

☐ Protein   ■ Fat   ☐ Starch Complex   ■ Sugar Simple

C a r b o h y d r a t e s

The American diet has been shifting, resulting in a dramatic change in diet composition, where now more calories come from sugar (simple carbohydrates) than from starch (complex carbohydrates) and almost half the calories come from fat. (US 1860-1990)

tables. They enjoyed hot cereals, cornbread, and biscuits. They ate rice, pasta, and corn, along with beans, potatoes, vegetables, and fruit. These nutritious high-fiber foods made up 53 percent of their daily calorie intake.

But times and tastes changed dramatically. Cereals like oatmeal have been replaced by cold, presweetened flakes. Lunch typically consists of a salad soaked in oily dressing, a hamburger, and a soda. Dinner often comes frozen in a cardboard box, or from the Colonel. Between meals there are sodas, chips, Ding Dongs, and donuts. Nutritious, high-fiber foods now represent only 22 percent of our daily calories, while fat consumption has nearly doubled and sugar intake has increased 240 percent.

That's frightening! What can be done?

Education is the key. As people learn that refinement robs food of most of its fiber and nutrients, and processing adds calories, subtracts nutrition, and contributes scores of chemical additives, many are willing to make changes.

People are also realizing that meat and dairy products should be used sparingly. While they carry nutrients, most are high in fat, cholesterol, and calories, and they contain virtually no fiber.

Today's people are increasingly giving up their preoccupation with rich animal products and processed foods and eating more complex carbohydrates—whole plant foods which are rich in fiber. Since 1970 the consumption of meat, whole milk, and eggs has decreased, and so has the number of heart attacks and strokes.

People know it, and science confirms it. The road to better health and longer life detours around fast-food outlets, feedlot animals, and shops full of contrived and depleted foods. Instead, the road leads us back to the gardens and farmlands of our country— the fresh fruits and crisp vegetables—and the kernels of golden grain.

Nutrition Chapter 4
Seven Wrong Roads

As Americans, we pride ourselves on being the best-fed nation on earth. But we are paying a high price for the privilege—in needless disease, disability, and premature death.

What are we doing wrong?

Americans are eating too much of nearly everything—too much sugar, too much fat, and too much salt. We eat too many calories. And we eat too often.

Such *abundance* has helped lay the foundation for coronary artery disease, stroke, high blood pressure, arthritis, adult onset diabetes, obesity, and several kinds of cancer. These diseases are responsible for three out of four deaths. They are related to lifestyle, especially to how we eat.

Disease from food? You must mean pesticides and preservatives!

Surprisingly, pesticides and preservatives aren't the worst offenders. Here are some of the more serious culprits:

• *Sugar.* The National Research Council reports that refined sugars and sweeteners account for up to 20 percent of many peo-

25

ple's daily calories. Devoid of fiber and nutrients, refined sugars are *empty,* or *naked,* calories. But because of their caloric density, they are well suited to promote obesity.

• *Refined Foods.* People used to think refinement was good because it got rid of *useless roughage.* Now we're learning how necessary fiber is in protecting us from certain cancers, stabilizing blood sugar, controlling weight, and preventing gastrointestinal problems such as gallstones, hemorrhoids, diverticulitis, and constipation.

• *Salt.* Most Westerners consume between 10 and 20 grams of salt a day (2 to 4 teaspoons). This is many times more than is actually needed and contributes prominently to high blood pressure, heart failure, and kidney disease.

• *Fat.* Most people don't realize that they are consuming about 36 percent to 40 percent of their daily calories as fat. This is much more than the body can properly handle. As a result, blood vessels plug up, causing coronary artery disease and strokes. A high fat diet also contributes to overweight, adult diabetes, and certain cancers.

• *Proteins.* A diet heavy in meat and animal products provides more protein, fat, and cholesterol than the body can use. Westerners eat two to three times more protein than is recommended. Scientists now recognize that a diet containing less protein, and much less fat and cholesterol, is essential for improved health and longevity.

• *Beverages.* North Americans seldom drink water. Instead, they average several servings of soda pop, beer, coffee, tea, and sweet drinks every day. Because most of these drinks are loaded with calories, yet lack fiber, they can play havoc with blood sugar levels and sabotage weight control efforts. Alcohol, caffeine, phosphates, and other chemicals found in beverages pose additional health risks.

• *Snacks.* Engineered taste sensations are taking the place of real food. Schools, day-care centers, even hospitals require snacks to be available. The coffee-break remains standard in work places as well as after-school and TV snacks at home. Well-planned family meals are now the exception. Snack attacks disrupt digestion and overburden the stomach, and are a frequent cause of bloating and indigestion.

Is there anything SAFE to eat?

Think fruit—hundreds of varieties, spectacular colors, and every imaginable texture and flavor. Also vegetables and tubers. In the legume family one finds scores of shapes, colors, and flavors. The grains present another gold mine of delectable and healthful foods.

People need to realize that eating a variety of whole-plant foods will furnish all the fat, protein, fiber, and nutrients the body needs. It is also ecologically sensitive and will cut the food budget in half.

The best news is that this kind of dietary lifestyle helps delay and often prevents the onset of most degenerative diseases. Not only does eating full-fiber plant foods allow people to eat larger quantities of food without having to worry about weight gain, but it promotes optimum health and energy for a lifetime.

Children

Getting Fatter
Faster

American children are getting fatter faster than ever. Four to six million youngsters aged 6 to 11 have serious weight problems, and the number of super-fat children has doubled during the last 15 years.

That's hard to believe. Isn't our culture more health conscious now? Aren't fitness clubs booming?

Physical fitness is a trend among adults, not children. It's grown-ups who are out running, walking, jogging, and joining fitness clubs and aerobic classes. It's the older people who flock to wellness lectures and examine menus at restaurants for healthier and leaner foods.

But don't schools have health courses, physical education, and sports activities?

Due to budget cuts, overcrowding, and teacher shortages, many schools have had to cut back on these programs in recent years. In some cases they've eliminated physical education courses and requirements altogether. Health classes are often unpop-

28

ular with students, and relatively few youngsters qualify for team positions in school-sponsored sports.

Isn't obesity in children mostly inherited?

Genes do play a role in a person's weight, but they aren't the whole answer. Environment plays a critically important role—as shown by the fact that the percentage of obese Americans has increased steadily over the past 50 years. Our gene pool can't change that fast!

We now have an environment that supports obesity. There was a time when children raced home from school to change clothes and go outside to play. They climbed trees, rode bicycles, skated, played games, and dribbled basketballs. Today's children average five to eight hours a day watching television!

What are the chances of a fat child becoming a fat adult?

About 80 percent of overweight teenagers will remain overweight as adults. The increase in adolescent obesity (about 40 percent during the last 15 years) will have serious consequences in the future.

Does obesity produce disease in childhood?

Being overweight predisposes a child to heart disease, gallstones, adult onset diabetes, hypertension, cancer, and full-blown obesity later in life. Obese children have more orthopedic problems and upper respiratory diseases. And that is only one side of the story. They often suffer major social and psychological problems. The rapid increase of serious depression, eating disorders, drug use, and suicide among teenagers is frightening.

What can be done about this growing problem?

The major causes of obesity in children are the same as for adults— a sedentary lifestyle, TV viewing, the snack and soda habit, and the popularity and availability of highly processed and concentrated foods. Many major medical centers are developing weight control programs for children that involve the whole family. Proper eating and lifestyle habits are a family affair, and a youngster especially needs the support of the family. Even when the rest of the family is not overweight everyone benefits from a healthier way of life.

Nearly all obesity in children could be prevented if children were taught the following sensible basic habits early, before they have free access to food and become addicted to TV:

- Three meals a day with lots of whole grains, legumes, fresh fruit, and vegetables, and no snacks or sodas between meals.

- Drink plenty of water.

- An hour or two of active exercise daily, preferably outdoors.

- Regular, quiet study and reading times to replace the hours spent watching TV.

- Plenty of rest. Many children are chronically tired. Put them to bed early enough so they awaken naturally, in time for a healthy breakfast.

- A wide range of interests—library visits, music lessons, arts and crafts, family outings, etc.

The Bible says—

"Train a child in the way he should go, and when he is old he will not turn from it."—Proverbs 22:6, NIV

Saving the child just might save the family.

Aging _____ Chapter 6
Older Can Be Better

Everyone hates getting old. People want to stay young, or at least middle-aged. But time keeps marching. With the *65 and older* segment getting larger in North America, what are the prospects for the golden-agers in today's world?

An increasing trend is to date people by their intellectual and social capabilities rather than by chronological age. Health, rather than years, usually determines one's status.

Old age sets in when disease and disability limit everyday tasks. Some people are old while still relatively young in years. These are usually people who are chronically ill, injured, or victims of a major tragedy, many of whom withdraw and give up on life. Others remain youthful and vital, interesting and productive into advanced age.

Some people claim older is better. Can that be?

It's a matter of perspective. For physical strength, energy, and fewer ailments, youth is better. But for increased confidence, better judgment and insight, less anxiety and more freedom, older can be better. And experience helps, too. Most philosophers, composers, painters, and writers, for instance, improve with time.

Don't most people over 65 suffer from chronic illnesses?

In affluent Western society, about 80 percent of the 65-and-over group have some kind of health problem such as high blood pressure, arthritis, or heart disease. But most of these illnesses are not incapacitating. About 95 percent of older people live in their communities, and most have their own households.

Premature aging and disability are largely the result of lifestyle factors such as smoking, excessive alcohol and caffeine consumption, and the abuse of drugs. Being overweight speeds up physical and sexual decline. A diet of rich, refined foods and lack of regular exercise can make people old before their time.

Isn't forgetfulness a bad sign?

Forgetfulness in older people is exaggerated. Stress, anxiety, fast-moving events, memory overload, and lack of interest can cause forgetfulness at any age. Depression, which affects many older people, is often misdiagnosed as senility. Only a few people develop Alzheimer's disease or other genuinely senile dementias. Most people retain remarkable memory function for a long time, especially when they stay active and fit.

Don't many older people end up in nursing homes?

Actually, in North America only two percent of people 64 to 75 years of age live in nursing homes. Only after age 85 does the figure reach 20 percent.

Today is a good time to be alive! Productive social activities are pushing back the aging process. So are exercise, a better understanding of the role of diet, earlier attention to health problems and advances in modern technology. People today are often staying physically and mentally fit into their 80s and 90s. Many remain sexually active as well.

There is more. Scientists are discovering that an optimistic, positive attitude actually boosts the body's immune mechanism. This sophisticated defense system is proving to be one of the major keys to good health.

The Good Book said it long ago: *"A merry heart does good, like medicine."*—Proverbs 17:22, NKJV

LIFESTYLE DISEASES

- *Heart Disease*
- *Reversing Heart Disease*
- *Hypertension*
- *Stroke*
- *Cancer*
- *Diabetes*
- *Osteoporosis*
- *Obesity*

Coronary Heart Disease — Chapter 7
Killer for Dinner

Hundreds of thousands of people die every year from heart attacks without a murmur of protest from the public, the press, or government agencies. Yet the nation's number one killer can be found right on the dinner table!

You mean, what we eat causes heart attacks?

Not everything. The main culprits are excessive amounts of fat and cholesterol. The underlying problem is a hardening, a plugging up of vital arteries that supply the heart with oxygen, a process known as atherosclerosis.

People are born with clean, flexible arteries which should stay that way throughout life. The arteries of many North Americans, however, are clogging up with cholesterol, fat, and calcium—a concoction which gradually hardens and eventually chokes off needed oxygen supplies.

During World War II most Europeans were forced to change their eating habits from their customary diet of meat, eggs, and dairy products to a more austere diet of potatoes, grains, beans, roots, and vegetables. The result? A dramatic decrease in atherosclerosis which lasted for several years.

Since then, massive amounts of data have accumulated from research on animals and humans around the world. The results are essentially the same: diets high in fat and cholesterol produce elevated levels of blood cholesterol and heart disease. Diets low in fat and cholesterol reduce blood cholesterol levels and heart disease and even permit plaque reversal.

How can I tell if I have atherosclerosis?

There simply aren't any hints of the problem until your arteries are seriously narrowed. Some people begin to experience angina (heart pain) on exertion. For many people a heart attack is the first sign of trouble. About one-third of heart attacks result in sudden death.

Who is at risk for heart attack?

The risk factor concept is a good way to determine the likelihood of coronary heart disease:

- The most serious risk factor by far is an elevated blood cholesterol. Fifty-year-old men with cholesterol levels over 295 mg% (or

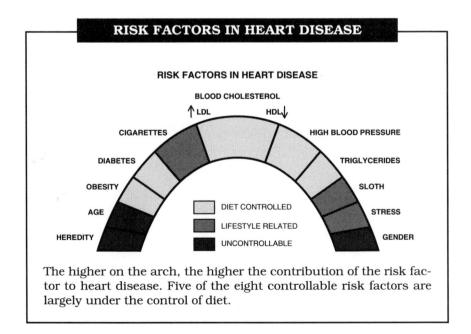

RISK FACTORS IN HEART DISEASE

RISK FACTORS IN HEART DISEASE

BLOOD CHOLESTEROL

↑LDL   HDL↓

CIGARETTES   HIGH BLOOD PRESSURE

DIABETES   TRIGLYCERIDES

OBESITY   SLOTH

AGE   DIET CONTROLLED   STRESS

LIFESTYLE RELATED

HEREDITY   UNCONTROLLABLE   GENDER

The higher on the arch, the higher the contribution of the risk factor to heart disease. Five of the eight controllable risk factors are largely under the control of diet.

7.6 mmol/L) are nine times more likely to develop atherosclerosis than men the same age with levels under 200 mg% (or 5.1 mmol/L). A 20 percent decrease in a person's blood cholesterol level lowers his risk of a coronary by 40 to 50 percent.

- By age 60, smokers are ten times more likely to die from heart disease than nonsmokers. Over 160,000 coronary deaths a year are related to smoking, about 30 percent of the total.

- In North America every third adult has high blood pressure, and is three times more likely to die of heart disease than a person with normal blood pressure.

- Obese men are five times more likely to die of heart disease by age 60 than men of normal weight.

- Other risk factors are diabetes, elevated triglycerides, sedentary lifestyle, and stress.

All of the above risk factors can be controlled by changes in diet and lifestyle. Heredity, age, and gender are risk factors a person cannot control, but they are fortunately the least important.

What about medications and surgery?

For those with dangerous cholesterol levels that do not respond adequately to diet, medications may be needed. Medications, however, are expensive and most have serious side effects. They require frequent laboratory tests and physician checkups.

More glamorous are the surgical procedures: bypass operations, roto-rooter cleanouts, and balloon stretching. Some results have been spectacular. But as time goes on and statistics accumulate, it is becoming apparent that most of these operations do not prolong life or even necessarily improve it. Medical treatment is temporary at best. The only long-term solution is a serious lifestyle change.

So what is the best approach?

The best possible approach is prevention, and it's never too late to start. But if heart disease has developed, as suggested by the presence of coronary risk factors and documented by diagnostic tests, it still isn't too late to make lifestyle changes. You can actually clean out your arteries, lower your risk of dying of atherosclerosis and extend your active, productive years. You can markedly change your risk factors no matter how old you are, often in just a few weeks.

Start with healthful, home-cooked meals that are very low in fat and cholesterol, yet high in unrefined complex carbohydrates and fiber. Such a diet can lower cholesterol levels by 20 percent to 30 percent and normalize most cases of adult diabetes in less than four weeks. When combined with salt restriction, this diet will also help normalize blood pressure and control obesity.

Begin an active, daily exercise program.

If Americans would lower their cholesterol to below 180, their blood pressures to under 125 and quit smoking, it has been estimated that 82 percent of all heart attacks before age 65 could be prevented. These simple changes in lifestyle would do more to improve the health of our nation than all the hospitals, surgeries, and drugs put together.

Eat Your Way Out

The sports world rejoiced when former Yale president, Dr. Bart Giamotti, became commissioner of baseball. A few months later a shocked nation wept when this respected man died suddenly at age 51, attacked by his heart.

Scenarios like this one are repeated thousands of times each day across North America. Heart disease now strikes a deadly blow to four out of every 10 Americans.

Is there a solution? Does it have to be like this?

Yes . . . and no.

As long as Americans continue to eat their rich, fatty diet, the statistics will remain the same. We've known for years that a high fat, high cholesterol diet is the primary cause of coronary heart disease.

But there is a solution: it requires that we *lean out* our high fat diet. To the extent that we do this, we can help prevent and even reverse heart disease.

Are you saying that heart disease may be curable?

It looks more and more that way.

The idea took on a life of its own when Dean Ornish, MD, published a report in the *LANCET* medical journal, in 1990, that shook up the medical community. Dr. Ornish spent one year studying 50 men with advanced heart disease, many of whom were candidates for coronary bypass surgery.

He randomly assigned the men to different groups. Both groups were asked to quit smoking and to walk daily. In addition, the first group practiced stress management and followed a vegetarian diet with less than 10 percent of calories as fat and no cholesterol.

The second group was given the American Heart Association's "Prudent Diet" for heart disease. This diet allowed 30 percent of calories as fat and up to 300 mg of cholesterol a day.

At the end of the year, when the results were presented at the Scientific Session of the American Heart Association in Washington, D.C., they became front page news all over America.

CALORIE CONCENTRATION: HOW FATS DO IT!

Food	Cal.	Empty Calories	Cal.	Total Calories
Lettuce and Tomato Salad	40 +	Roquefort dressing	160	200
Whole Wheat Bread (1 slice)	65 +	Butter	70	135
Broccoli (1/2 cup)	35 +	Cheese Sauce	130	165
Vegetarian Entree or Broiled Fish (6 oz.)	220 +	Tartar Sauce	80	300
Large Baked Potato with Salsa	135 +	Sour Cream and Butter	180	315
Skim Milk (1 glass)	90 or	Whole Milk		160
Baked Apple with date or walnut	100 or	Apple Pie a la mode (1/6)		500
Total Calories	**685**		**Total Calories**	**1,775**

Dr. Ornish reported that those on the very low-fat vegetarian diet not only dropped their average blood cholesterol level by 40 percent, but their narrow, plaque-filled arteries had actually widened, allowing more blood and oxygen to the heart muscle. The heart disease had, in fact, begun to reverse itself. And the older men with the more advanced disease actually had the best results.

The group on the so-called "Prudent Diet," however, had virtually no cholesterol drop, and their coronary arteries showed increased narrowing. Their heart disease had actually gotten worse.

You mean the American Heart Association's diet did not help at all?

It appears that the "Prudent Diet" designed for the prevention and treatment of heart disease does not do its job. At the press conference Dr. Ornish concluded: "The moderate diet recommendations of the American Heart Association do not go far enough to effectively influence the progression of coronary heart disease. People with clinically demonstrated disease need to go beyond the present dietary recommendation."

We have known for years that much of today's heart disease could be prevented, but it's exciting to realize that, under the proper conditions, it is possible to reverse it. This revolutionary study suggests that, given the proper diet, we may be able to eat ourselves out of heart disease.

Hypertension   Chapter 9
The Silent
Killer

Every third adult in North America has high blood pressure. These hypertensives are three times more likely to have a heart attack, five times more likely to develop heart failure, and eight times more likely to suffer a stroke than are people with normal blood pressure.

How can I know if I have hypertension?

Hypertension is defined as a systolic blood pressure reading (the top number) consistently over 140, and/or a diastolic (lower number) reading of 90 or above. Even though there are no symptoms (that's why it is called the *silent disease*), such conditions cause progressive changes in the blood vessels until the first sign hits, usually a stroke or a heart attack.

What causes the blood pressure to go up?

Certain kinds of tumors will do it, also diseases within the kidney itself. But in 90 percent of everyday hypertension, the specific organic cause cannot be determined. This kind of hypertension is called *essential* hypertension.

The following factors contribute to essential hypertension:

- *High Salt Intake.* Surprisingly, hypertension is uncommon in 80 percent of the world's population. Salt intake is low in these areas. In places where salt intake is high, as in Japan, the disease is epidemic, affecting approximately one half of adults. Americans consume an average of 10 to 20 grams of salt per day. That's two to four teaspoonfuls or about 10-20 times more than the body needs!

- *Obesity.* Nearly everyone who is significantly overweight will eventually experience high blood pressure. It's just a matter of time.

- *Arterial Plaque.* Narrowed and plugged arteries force the body to boost the blood pressure in order to deliver necessary oxygen and food to body cells.

- *Estrogen.* This hormone, found in birth control pills and used to ease menopausal symptoms, is also a salt retainer. It can raise blood pressure by holding excess fluid in the body.

- *Alcohol.* Scientific studies have demonstrated that alcohol intake accounts for 5 percent to 15 percent of cases of ordinary hypertension.

Why do Americans eat so much salt?

In today's life it's hard to get away from salt. About 75 percent of our salt intake comes from fast and processed foods. A taste for salt is easy to develop, and salty snacks and foods abound to accommodate us.

What about medications for hypertension?

The past few years have produced an avalanche of new drugs that are effective in lowering blood pressure. Some are lifesaving. Most produce prompt results—the quick fix that Americans love.

But a closer look at hypertension medications reveals some disquieting facts: the drugs do not cure hypertension, they only control it. In many cases the medications need to be taken for life. Unpleasant side effects may include fatigue, depression, and lack of sexual desire. While the drugs help protect against strokes, they do not protect against coronary atherosclerosis (the plugging of heart arteries). They may actually *promote* atherosclerosis, diabetes, and gouty arthritis.

What are the alternatives?

A number of major scientific studies have shown that simple dietary and lifestyle changes can reverse most essential hypertension in a matter of weeks without drugs.

- A large percentage of people are sensitive to salt and would benefit from its reduction in their diets.
- When the weight goes down blood pressure levels usually fall. Reducing excess weight is often the only treatment needed to correct a rising blood pressure.
- A low-fat, high-fiber diet lowers the blood pressure about 10 percent even without weight loss or salt restriction. Thinning of the blood, which results from eating less fat, probably produces these favorable changes.
- Deleting alcohol from the diet will lower blood pressure and do the body a favor in several other areas as well.
- Physical exercise lowers blood pressure by reducing peripheral arterial resistance. In addition, regular exercise promotes general health and well-being.

People taking blood pressure medications should not play *doctor* and change doses or stop medicines on their own. But those who are willing to make healthful lifestyle changes will usually find their physicians glad to help them eat and exercise their way out of hypertension.

Stroke Chapter 10
Stalking a Crippler

Two million Americans lie crippled from paralyzing strokes. After AIDS and cancer, stroke is probably the most dreaded and disabling disease to afflict Westernized civilizations.

What are a person's chances of developing a stroke?

Half a million Americans have strokes each year. As with heart attacks, serious and even fatal strokes can occur without warning. Around one-fourth of victims under age 70 die from the first attack; after that the figure doubles.

Of those who survive, 40 percent need some degree of on-going special care, but only 10 percent require institutionalization.

The remaining 60 percent represent the good news. Some recover completely; nearly all improve enough to care for themselves; most are able to resume their normal activities.

What causes strokes?

A stroke, or Cerebral Vascular Accident (CVA), is most commonly related to atherosclerosis—a thickening, narrowing, and hardening of arteries supplying the brain with oxygenated blood. This atherosclerotic process can occur both in arteries within the brain and

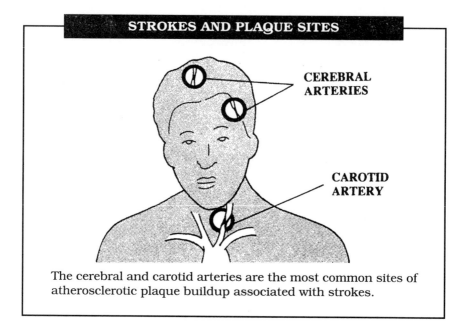

STROKES AND PLAQUE SITES

CEREBRAL ARTERIES

CAROTID ARTERY

The cerebral and carotid arteries are the most common sites of atherosclerotic plaque buildup associated with strokes.

in arteries leading to the brain. The roughened, ragged inner surfaces of damaged arteries become seedbeds for clot formation and plaque buildup. When obstruction is complete, the artery is said to be *thrombosed.*

Sometimes pieces of plaque or a blood clot break off from other parts of the circulatory system and travel to smaller brain arteries, producing obstruction. These are called *emboli.* Some 85 percent of CVAs result from either thrombotic or embolic arterial blockage.

Hemorrhages, or blowouts, cause the rest of the strokes. Most of these are associated with uncontrolled high blood pressure which forces blood through cracks in stiffened artery walls. A few blowouts are caused by *aneurysms.* These are ballooned-out areas in certain arteries which get thinner and thinner until they rupture. The result, either way, is bleeding into the brain.

Strokes do their damage by preventing fresh blood from reaching an area of the brain, which soon dies from lack of oxygen. If a large portion of the brain is affected, the stroke will be severe or fatal. A smaller area of brain damage will cause lesser symptoms.

Who is at risk for strokes?

Most strokes are directly related to high blood pressure. People with hypertension are eight times more likely to suffer a stroke than are people with normal blood pressure.

Blackout spells, called *Transient Ischemic Attacks* (TIAs) may be early warnings. These are small strokes which start suddenly and disappear in less than 24 hours. Most last only a few seconds, and recovery is complete. Persistent TIAs, however, increase the chances for a complete stroke, much as angina attacks increase the chances of a heart attack.

Other risk factors include elevated blood cholesterol and triglycerides, smoking, diabetes, obesity, and sedentary lifestyle, all of which contribute to the atherosclerotic process. In fact, the risk factors for stroke are basically the same as those for coronary heart disease, because both diseases are caused by underlying damage to vital, oxygen-carrying arteries.

Can strokes be prevented?

Yes, most strokes can be prevented. In fact strokes, like certain other lifestyle diseases, could become relatively uncommon within a generation if people would begin adopting, early in life, the healthful lifestyle practices already known today. These include the following:

- Don't smoke. One out of every six CVA deaths is directly related to tobacco use.
- Check blood pressure regularly. Hypertension has no symptoms, and it can sneak up on the unaware. Remember, hypertension increases a person's stroke risk by 800 percent.
- Learn to use much less salt. In areas of the world where salt intake is low, hypertension is virtually unknown. In Japan, where salt intake is high, stroke is the leading cause of death.

- Normalize weight. Obesity promotes atherosclerosis, hypertension, and most diabetes.
- Eat a low-fat, low-cholesterol, high-fiber diet. Keeping fat intake to less than 20 percent of daily calories has been shown to protect arterial linings from atherosclerosis.
- Exercise actively and regularly. Exercise improves circulation and helps control weight and hypertension.

What about people who've already had strokes? Is there help for them?

Definitely. The lifestyle that helps prevent strokes will also hasten recovery, as well as help prevent recurrent strokes.

Acute strokes require good nursing care and energetic rehabilitation. In selected cases, surgical procedures such as endarterectomy (cleaning out the arteries) are of value.

Small doses of aspirin have been shown to help prevent strokes in susceptible people. Remember, however, that aspirin may also promote bleeding tendencies and aggravate stomach ulcers.

But the best news is that arterial blockages are reversible. Thickened, narrowed arteries slowly open again when a *very* low-fat, vegetarian diet is consistently followed, along with the other health practices. While these studies, so far, center on coronary arteries, similar results are expected in arteries affecting the brain, since the underlying problem is the same.

For proof that these principles work, look at stroke statistics in the United States and Canada. With advances in the treatment of hypertension, and improved diet and lifestyle practices, the incidence of strokes has declined over 50 percent during the last 30 years.

Everyone is born with soft, flexible, elastic artery walls. Many populations around the world retain their healthy arteries and low blood pressures throughout their lifetimes. We can, too, if we get serious about pursuing healthful lifestyle practices before the damage is done.

Cancer | *Chapter 11*

Do-It-Yourself Cancers

Many cancers are turning out to be do-it-yourself diseases. We promote them by chronic exposure to certain environmental factors. What we eat and drink, where we live and work, and what we breathe may well determine whether we become a cancer statistic.

Are you saying that we bring cancer on ourselves?

Medical science continues to make strides toward earlier detection and improved treatments for many cancers. But these efforts are largely *after the fact*. The sad truth is that the overall death rates for many cancers continue to rise. One in four American lives are now being claimed by cancer.

This trend, however, could be reversed. If we would simply take the precautions that we already know about, 70 percent to 80 percent of the cancers that afflict Americans could be prevented.

Won't people do just about anything to avoid *such a terrifying disease?*

Almost anything, it seems, except change their lifestyles.

Take lung cancer, for example; the cancer that kills more men

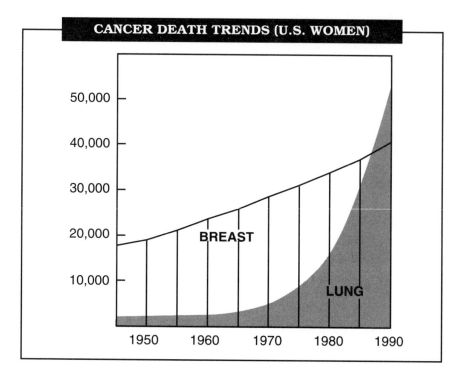

CANCER DEATH TRENDS (U.S. WOMEN)

and women in the United States than any other. Ever since the Surgeon General's report in 1964 we've known that lung cancer is directly related to cigarette smoking. It's true that millions have quit smoking, yet every fourth adult in North America still smokes! Close to 90 percent of the cancers of the lung, lip, mouth, tongue, throat, and esophagus could be prevented if people simply stopped using tobacco. It would also prevent half the bladder cancers.

Are some cancers related to diet?

In men, the second and third most frequently occurring cancers are those of the prostrate and colon. For women it's cancers of the breast and colon. Extensive evidence links nearly 50 percent of these cancers to over-nutrition—too much fat and too much weight.

How about chemicals and pesticides?

Carcinogens (cancer-producing chemicals) are a concern, especially with the array of additives, preservatives, flavor enhancers, pesticides, and other chemicals that we use in producing and marketing food. However, only 2 percent of all cancers can be reliably linked to these substances.

In contrast, evidence of the connection between cancer and such dietary factors as fiber and fat grows stronger every day. Compared with diets at the turn of the century, the average American now eats 36 percent *more* fat, and one-third *less* fiber. In areas of the world where fat intake is low and fiber consumption is high, there is a negligible incidence of colon, breast, and prostate cancers. In countries such as the United States, Canada, and New Zealand, where diets are low in fiber and high in fat, rates for these kinds of cancers are much higher.

Could racial variations, rather than diet, account for these differences?

Researchers have asked the same question. They have found, for example, that Japanese living in villages and rural areas have very few of these cancers. Their traditional fiber consumption is high, and fat intake averages only 15 percent to 20 percent of the diet. But when Japanese migrate to America and adopt Western eating habits and lifestyles, their rates for these cancers increase dramatically and soon equal those for Americans.

How can such things as fiber and fat influence cancer?

Not all the answers are in yet, but cancer is associated with carcinogens—chemical irritants that can produce cancerous lesions over time.

Bile acids are an example. The amount of fat in the diet affects the amount of bile the body produces. In the intestinal tract some of these bile acids can form irritating carcinogenic compounds. The longer these compounds stay in contact with the lining of the colon the more irritation results.

This is where fiber comes in. With a low-fiber diet, material moves slowly through the intestines, often taking from 72 hours to seven days to complete the journey from entry to exit. Fiber absorbs water like a sponge. This helps fill the intestines and stimulates them to increased activity. With a high-fiber diet food travels through the intestines in 24 to 36 hours.

This helps the colon in two ways. It shortens the exposure to irritating substances, and it dilutes the concentration of the irritants because of fiber's water-holding ability and insulating effect.

What about other cancers?

A high fat intake depresses the activity of important cells in the body's immune system. This effect has been studied extensively in connection with breast cancer and may well affect other types of cancer as well.

Excessive alcohol consumption increases the risk for cancer of the esophagus and pancreas, and does so dramatically for those who smoke as well. Excess weight raises the risk of cancer of the breast, colon, and prostate. Then there are such things as exposure to asbestos, sidestream smoke, and toxic chemicals.

Just four lifestyle factors—no smoking, no alcohol, a high-fiber, low-fat vegetarian diet, and normal weight—could prevent close to 75 percent of cancers found in Western society today. Instead of one American in four dying of cancer, the risk could be reduced to one in 20.

It's not an impossible dream.

Diabetes   Chapter 12

Disarming Diabetes

n times past a diagnosis of diabetes was somewhat akin to one
of leprosy: once you got it, it stuck around for the duration. And
it brought along a lifetime of loathsome burdens.

No more! Today many people are beating diabetes. They are normalizing their blood sugars and getting off insulin by making
healthful lifestyle changes.

What exactly is diabetes? And isn't it inherited?

Diabetes occurs when the body becomes unable to handle glucose
(sugar) which builds up to dangerous levels in the blood. The problem
revolves around insulin, a pancreatic hormone that enables body
cells to use glucose and thus brings down high blood sugar levels.

There are two kinds of diabetes. Type I afflicts about 5 percent
of diabetics. They are usually thin and rarely overweight. This
type of diabetes is often hereditary, usually begins in childhood or
youth and is commonly called *juvenile diabetes.* Since these diabetics cannot survive without insulin, it is now officially called
Insulin Dependent Diabetes Mellitus (IDDM).

Type II diabetes is different. Called "adult onset diabetes," or *Non-
Insulin Dependent Diabetes* (NIDDM), it afflicts an estimated 15 mil-

TYPES OF DIABETES

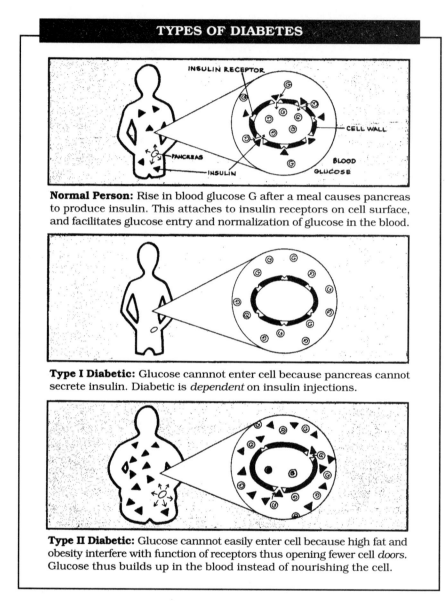

Normal Person: Rise in blood glucose G after a meal causes pancreas to produce insulin. This attaches to insulin receptors on cell surface, and facilitates glucose entry and normalization of glucose in the blood.

Type I Diabetic: Glucose cannnot enter cell because pancreas cannot secrete insulin. Diabetic is *dependent* on insulin injections.

Type II Diabetic: Glucose cannnot easily enter cell because high fat and obesity interfere with function of receptors thus opening fewer cell *doors*. Glucose thus builds up in the blood instead of nourishing the cell.

lion Americans. This type generally hits after age 50 as people get older and fatter. In contrast to the juvenile diabetics, most Type II diabetics, when diagnosed, have plenty of insulin in their bodies. But something blocks the insulin; it cannot do its job.

What causes Type II diabetes?

Studies demonstrate a strong relationship to fat, both fat in the diet and fat on the body. The disease is rare in areas of the world where fat intake is low and obesity uncommon.

Most of the time the problem in adult onset diabetes is not a defective pancreas unable to produce sufficient insulin, but a lack of sensitivity to insulin. This resistance of the cells to insulin appears to relate directly to obesity and to excess fat in the diet.

But isn't sugar the culprit?

James Anderson, MD, professor of medicine and clinical nutrition at the University of Kentucky Medical College and a respected authority on diabetes, evaluated the effect of diet composition on blood sugar levels. Just as others had done before him, Dr. Anderson was able to turn lean, healthy young men into mild diabetics in less than two weeks by feeding them a rich 65 percent fat diet. A similar group, fed a lean 10 percent fat diet plus one pound of sugar per day, did not produce even one diabetic after 11 weeks when the experiment was terminated.

So what's the best way to treat this disease?

Several treatment centers have convincingly demonstrated that *most* Type II diabetics can normalize their blood sugar levels, often within weeks, by following a simple diet, very low in fat and high in fiber, coupled with daily exercise.

Lowering the amount of fat, oil, and grease in the diet plays a crucial role. When less fat is eaten, less fat reaches the bloodstream. This begins a complicated process which gradually *unblocks* the insulin, which can then facilitate the entry of sugar from the bloodstream into the body cells. The effect is often dramatic. A Type II diabetic who lowers daily fat intake down to 10 percent to 15 percent of total calories can often bring blood sugar levels to normal ranges in less than eight weeks. Many are eventually able to get off diabetic medication entirely—both pills and injections.

Eating more natural, fiber-rich foods plays an important role by helping stabilize blood sugar levels. When foods are eaten without their normal complement of fiber, blood sugar levels can shoot up. Normally a surge of insulin counteracts this. People who consume refined foods, drinks, and snacks high in calories but low in fiber may experience hikes and dips in blood sugar levels all day long. High fiber foods, on the other hand, smooth out these blood sugar fluctuations and stabilize energy levels.

Active physical exercise has an insulin-like reaction in that it *burns up the fuel* (blood sugar and fatty acids) more rapidly.

Normalizing body weight is often all that is necessary to bring the blood sugar back to normal. The low-fat, high-fiber diet will greatly aid this effort, as will regular, active exercise.

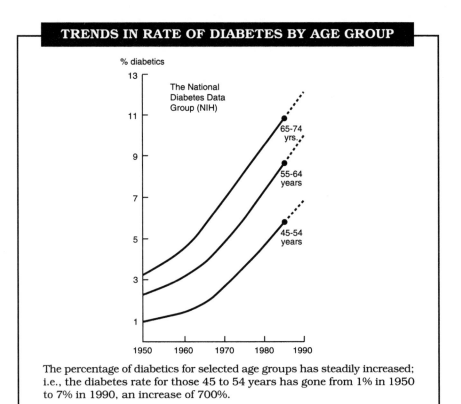

TRENDS IN RATE OF DIABETES BY AGE GROUP

% diabetics

The National Diabetes Data Group (NIH)

65-74 yrs.

55-64 years

45-54 years

The percentage of diabetics for selected age groups has steadily increased; i.e., the diabetes rate for those 45 to 54 years has gone from 1% in 1950 to 7% in 1990, an increase of 700%.

What about Type I diabetes?

Insulin dependent, or juvenile diabetics, will need to take insulin for life until pancreatic transplants become accessible. However, the high-fiber, low-fat diet can help reduce the amount of insulin required to maintain stable blood sugar levels and reduce the ever present threat of vascular complications.

Today, a newborn baby who lives 70 years, will have a one-in-five chance of becoming diabetic, if the present diabetic rate trends continue, according to the National Institutes of Health. But this need not be! The same lifestyle measures that are disarming and normalizing many cases of Type II diabetes are preventive as well. Start now. Beat diabetes before it happens!

Osteoporosis   Chapter 13
Building Better Bones

What is osteoporosis?

Osteoporosis (literally, *porous bone*) silently and painlessly weakens the bones of 25 million Americans. Previously sturdy bones gradually become thin and fragile, their interiors soft and spongy. As a result, bones break, giving rise to the term *brittle bones.*

Osteoporosis may cause as many as 1.3 million fractures a year. Hip fractures can be both disabling and deadly. Spinal fractures, on the other hand, are often painless, but can rob a person of two to eight inches of height. The resultant spinal curvature is the source of *dowager's hump.*

How can I tell if I have it?

Without professional help, you can't—not until you fracture a bone or start shrinking in height, and that's very late in the disease. Earlier diagnosis is best done by physicians at reliable medical centers.

If you are middle-aged or older, and have two or more of the following risk factors, you should be tested:

- sedentary lifestyle
- high-protein diet
- low estrogen
- early menopause
- chronic use of corticosteroids
- cigarettes, caffeine, or alcohol

Lean Caucasians and Asians are more susceptible than other races probably because they have smaller bones.

How does osteoporosis develop?

Normal bones continue to increase in strength and thickness until around age 35. Then the process gradually reverses itself, and small amounts of bone are lost each year. This loss accelerates in women after menopause and can continue for seven to 15 years. When risk factors are present, bone loss occurs even faster and osteoporosis may develop.

Although usually considered a disease of older women, 20 percent of victims are men.

What can be done to treat this disease?

Several treatments are being used:

• *Estrogen therapy:* When used, it slows down bone loss, but increases the risk for uterine and breast cancer, thrombophlebitis (blood clots) and gallbladder disease. It aggravates diabetes and hypertension. Women also face the prospect of continuing menstrual periods and periodic uterine biopsies. In high risk cases, however, the benefits may outweigh the risks.

• *Vitamin D:* The body uses vitamin D to absorb calcium, but most Americans get more than they need and additional supplements have not proven beneficial.

• *Fluoride:* It is used experimentally, but long-term results are controversial.

• *Calcium:* The World Health Organization recommends 500 mg of calcium a day, while various health organizations in North America recommend 800 to 1,500 mg. These dosages may be prudent for some; however, most studies of world populations show little or no correlation between calcium intake and bone density.

• *Exercise:* Bones will not thicken and strengthen without regular, weight-bearing exercise, such as walking. To retain their minerals, bones *need* to be pressed, pushed, pulled, and twisted against gravity.

The gravity factor was well demonstrated by the early astronauts. Even though they exercised faithfully while in space, their bones showed startling osteoporotic changes on their return. While nearly all types of aerobic exercise are beneficial to the body, what the bones need most is a good daily shake-up.

• *A low protein diet:* This is the most promising therapy on the horizon. The body uses calcium in its metabolism of excess protein and then flushes the calcium out the kidneys. Studies show that calcium is always lost from bones when protein intake is too high—regardless of how many calcium-rich foods one eats or how many calcium supplements one swallows.

What makes you think protein might be a culprit?

Eskimos in the far north consume diets extremely high in both protein (250 to 400 gm/day) and calcium (1,500 to 2,500 mg/day). In spite of their high calcium intake and the very active lives they lead, they have the highest rate of osteoporosis of any world population.

The Bantu tribes in Africa, on the other hand, consume an average of 47 grams of protein and less than 400 mg of calcium a day, predominantly from plant foods. Yet, even though Bantu women bear an average of 10 or more children, making special demands on calcium reserves, they are essentially free of osteoporosis. In contrast, relatives of the Bantu who have migrated to the United States and adopted the American dietary lifestyle eventually experience a rate of osteoporosis comparable to that of the rest of the American population.

How about prevention?

Most populations around the world average 200 to 400 mg of calcium a day without evidence of osteoporosis. It's strangely paradoxical that osteoporosis has become epidemic in the United

States, where the consumption of calcium-rich dairy products and calcium supplements is the highest in the world.

North Americans eat two to three times more protein than they need. Reducing protein intake to the Recommended Daily Allowance of 50- 60 grams per day, along with daily active exercise and a healthful diet, holds promise of turning the tide in the battle against brittle bones.

HOW EASY IT IS TO EAT TOO MUCH PROTEIN!

Breakfast	Protein (gm)	
3-egg ham and cheese omelette	46	
Hash brown potatoes	3	
Toast (2) with butter and jelly	5	
Coffee with cream	1	
Orange juice	1	
Lunch		
Big Mac	26	
French fries	3	
Milkshake	11	
Dinner		
Fried chicken	55	
Peas	5	
Mixed salad with dressing	4	
Baked potato with sour cream	9	**TOTAL**
Milk (2%), 1 glass	9	**178 gms**

Chapter 14

Creeping Fat

Americans, on the average, are heavier than the citizens of any other major nation. Obesity is one of our leading public health problems. So serious is this disease that 36 million people are at significant medical risk.

That's frightening. No wonder weight-loss diets *are so popular!*

Yes, and far too many people fall prey to fads and eating plans that offer quick results. Like a conditioned reflex, extra pounds spell d-i-e-t to most people. A recent survey found that 40 percent to 50 percent of Americans between the ages of 35 and 59 were on some kind of diet at any given time.

The sad truth is that unless people make lasting changes in their lifestyles and consistently choose healthful foods on a regular basis, their efforts are largely wasted. Up to 90 percent of dieters regain their lost weight within a year, usually with a bonus. Constantly losing and regaining weight is frustrating and demoralizing, and does more damage than good.

Would it be better to just stay fat?

For many people, remaining overweight would be less harmful than endlessly playing the rhythm game of *girth control.* Before running up the white flag of surrender, however, take a careful look at the health risks of being overweight.

Extra weight shortens life. Recent reports indicate that as little as five to 10 pounds increase mortality figures. It's been calculated that every extra pound shaves about one month from one's lifespan. Sixty pounds will cost five years!

Obesity, by definition, occurs when a person is 20 percent or more above ideal weight. Being 10 percent to 19 percent over ideal weight is usually termed overweight.

Excess weight lays the foundation for nearly every degenerative disease except osteoporosis. Obese people are three times more likely to have heart disease, four times more likely to suffer from high blood pressure, five times more likely to develop diabetes and elevated blood cholesterols, and six times more likely to have gallbladder disease. They also develop more cancer of the colon, rectum, prostate, breast, cervix, uterus, and ovaries, and suffer more osteoarthritis and low back pain. Overweight people are like ticking bombs waiting for one or more of these diseases to explode in their lives.

In addition, extra weight affects self image. In today's appearance-oriented society it can be a great psychological burden.

How do extra pounds harm the body?

The key to the problem is calories—too many of them. Overweight happens when you eat more calories than your body can use. Whether calories come from fat, protein, sugar, or starch, the leftovers are turned into fat. Some of this fat floats around in the blood, plastering and gradually plugging vital oxygen-carrying arteries.

The rest of the leftover fat ends up in the body's central fat bank, located around the midsection. Embarrassing branch offices often pop up in other parts of the body. For every 3,500 excess calories received by the body, one pound of fat is placed on deposit.

Excess fat relates directly to health. A 10 percent weight *reduction* in men 35 to 55 years of age will result in a 20 percent decrease in coronary heart disease. On the other hand, a 10 percent *increase* in weight produces a 30 percent increase in coronary disease. This is just one example of many such relationships. Every pound counts, one way or the other.

So what's the secret of lasting weight loss?

The strategy for successful weight control is threefold:

- Increase the quality and amount of food eaten while decreasing the number of calories.
- Increase the rate at which calories are burned by increasing physical activity and muscle size.
- Make the above two lifestyle practices a permanent part of life.

Begin by eating generous amounts of high-fiber foods, like whole grains, vegetables, fruits, potatoes, yams, and beans. Omit as much fat and sugar from the diet as possible, as well as refined and processed foods and snacks. These things are stuffed with calories and have negligible nutrients.

Use animal products such as meat, eggs, ice cream, and cheese very sparingly. They have no fiber and are loaded with fat.

This kind of eating plan, plus a brisk daily walk, will help you lose one to two pounds a week.

You can fight creeping fat, push up your energy level, improve your digestion, and feel good every day. Beginning right now!

WEIGHT CONTROL

- *Myths and Fads*
- *Diets*
- *Soft Drinks*
- *Snacks*
- *Exercise*
- *Calories*
- *Ideal Weight*
- *Fail-Safe Formula*

Myths and Fads   Chapter 15

When Success Is an Illusion

The appeal is all but irresistible. LOSE 10 POUNDS IN 10 DAYS— *with a new, scientifically proven formula!* The struggling, discouraged, overweight person grasps for another straw. He needs to believe.

Weight loss is weight loss, isn't it? Does it matter how a person loses it?

Most people who lose weight believe they are losing fat; in reality they may be losing mostly water plus muscle and other vital tissues.

Several years ago diet pills were popular. Many of them included a diuretic (water pill). Since the body is about 70 percent water it is relatively easy for such pills to remove several pounds of water quickly. The scales look good—for a few days. But gradually the body balances itself by replacing the water, and there goes the weight loss.

An overdose of protein will accomplish basically the same result. The liver changes excess protein into blood urea nitrogen (BUN) which causes the kidneys to force water from the body. It takes much more water to wash out the products of excess protein metabolism than it does to take care of the breakdown products of either carbohydrates or fats.

Some quick weight loss diets take advantage of the fact that a high protein intake can cause spectacular weight loss in a short time. This is a dangerous practice, however. That's why such diets are usually physician-supervised and limited to short periods of time, normally about two weeks. The scales show gratifyingly low numbers, but most of the weight returns in a short time as the body replaces lost water.

What other possible problems can such diets cause?

Many of the *quickie* diets drop daily calorie intake to extremely low levels—500 to 800 calories a day. Some even go as low as 300 to 400 calories. The body misreads this dramatic calorie drop as *acute starvation* and actually begins to digest its own protein (usually in the form of muscle) in an effort to protect more vital tissues. Careful testing has shown that weight loss on these diets can come from both fat and muscle tissues.

So beware! When you think you are losing 14 pounds of fat, for example, you could actually be losing five pounds of fat, one pound of protein tissue (muscle) and eight pounds of water.

If you feel you need to go on a diet, make sure calorie intake contains not only enough protein for daily needs but also enough carbohydrate to prevent muscle tissue loss. For an average person this means at least 200 calories of protein (50 grams) and 600 to 800 calories of carbohydrate a day. The body cannot use fat (fatty acids) for 100 percent of its fuel needs.

Can I really lose weight on such a gradual diet?

Moderately overweight people usually lose one to two pounds a week on a well-balanced diet; seriously overweight persons may lose a little more. Slow, steady weight loss has many advantages over the radical diets: it does not throw the body into the mode of *starvation metabolism,* binges and failures are much less frequent, hunger becomes more manageable, and chances are good that the weight lost is really fat.

But perhaps the most important aspect of slower weight loss is that it allows time to establish new and more healthful habits of eating. A person must develop a lifestyle that is consistent with maintaining the new weight if the weight loss is to have any chance of being permanent.

I'm desperate to lose weight; I have no patience with slow programs. Wouldn't quick weight loss be better than none at all?

Losing and regaining weight, over and over, is one of the most harmful things you can do to your body. The truth is that remaining overweight would be less harmful to overall health than this yo-yo effect. Repeated weight loss through crash diets, followed by regaining the weight, gradually depletes muscle tissue and adds fat tissue. And because muscle tissue is where fat is burned, you will become increasingly unable to lose weight.

Of even more concern are the psychological consequences. Enduring years of repeated failure and humiliation produces emotional scars that often remain for a lifetime. People seduced by the magic of quick weight loss offered by the merchants of misery, do shed pounds initially, but they almost invariably end up weighing more than they did before.

This is not to minimize the fact that overweight persons carry increased health risks. They have more heart disease, hypertension, diabetes, gallbladder disease, and cancer than do people of normal weight. They also die sooner.

Don't become a slave to the scale, checking it daily for immediate results to problems that took years to develop. Get started on a healthful program. And be patient. It's the long haul that matters. The illusions will fade, but the eventual rewards will be solid and lasting.

Diets

Chapter 16
The Quick-Fix Trap

We spend billions of dollars every year on diets and weight control paraphernalia, yet the results are dismal. For many, permanent, successful weight control is more difficult to achieve than victory over drugs, tobacco or alcohol.

Would it be better to stop trying? To just stay fat?

Yes, it would be safer to remain obese than to jump from one diet fad to another, lose pounds now, and gain them back later. Research shows that this yo-yo effect gradually depletes important body tissues such as muscle and bone. Eventually it weakens the body so that it becomes more susceptible to disease and less able to shed excess fat.

But isn't it dangerous to remain overweight?

Being fat isn't healthful. Excess weight impairs health and shortens life. As little as 10 to 15 pounds of extra weight produces measurable changes that can lay the foundation for degenerative disease. And for every 10 pounds of overweight, a lifespan can be shortened by as much as a year.

So what is the answer?

People who are overweight need major revisions in thinking and attitudes. The scenario played out in millions of lives goes something like this: a few weeks on the latest wonder diet; have the jaws wired; take a series of shots or pills; check into a fat farm. And presto, down goes the weight! Celebration! New clothes!

But within days these people resume their former eating patterns and lifestyle. In a few weeks or months the lost pounds are back, often with a bonus.

Weight control programs usually fail because they are short-term fixes for long-term problems. It's time to face the reality that obesity can be a serious and life-threatening condition.

OK, I'm convinced. What must I do?

Managing obesity is much more than a dietary problem. Like diabetes, hypertension, alcoholism, or smoking, obesity requires a comprehensive approach to lifestyle changes.

First, you have to have a long-term commitment, a life-long commitment that does not change when binges or other serious lapses occur. With this kind of commitment, you can get up when you fall, start again, and persevere.

Second, you need to identify and change habits that cause obesity. This may be as simple as eliminating soft drinks or cutting back on fats and oils. Or it may require you to completely restructure your eating patterns and lifestyle.

Changing lifelong habits is among the most difficult things a person can do, and the process is very threatening. Faithful, regular meetings with a support group greatly increases the chances of success. This kind of team effort is almost a *must* for those more than 20 pounds overweight or who have had problems several years.

Third, attitudes often need radical surgery. *Willingness* to change is critically important. Read books, attend seminars, join fitness groups, and make friends with health-minded people. Weight control is not a vanity trip. Keep the focus on improved health, and the weight will take care of itself.

Finally, look for a weight-control plan that is consistent with a lifetime of good health. This will include regular exercise, a low-fat, high-fiber diet, and a physical, mental, and psychological outlook that meets your needs in every area of life. Weight control should be only part of a full and fulfilling life—not its main preoccupation.

Such a workable life plan is possible. Many have succeeded. Put your heart into it and keep it there.

> *"Whatever your hand finds to do, do it with all your might."*
> —Ecclesiastes 9:10, NIV

Soft Drinks   Chapter 17

Carbonated Generation

Americans now drink more soft drinks than water. We average two soft drinks per day for every man, woman, and child in the country. Many people are concerned about possible health implications.

Aren't soft drinks a good way to help people drink *more fluids?*

Take one glass of water, add eight to 12 teaspoons of sugar, mix in a dose of chemicals—and you'll get a soft drink.

The extra sugar intake from soft drinks produces at least five undesirable side effects:

• *Unbalanced nutrition.* Most soft drinks contain 120 to 180 calories of sugar, but no needed nutrients. A typical sedentary woman requires only about 1,200 to 1,600 total calories a day to maintain optimal weight and good health. Two or three soft drinks can considerably reduce her daily food allotment as well as her nutrient supply. Over time, this imbalance could cause her nutritional status to become marginal.

The same applies to sedentary men who need about 1,600 to 2,400 calories a day.

HOW MANY CALORIES DO YOU *DRINK* IN A DAY?		
Drink	**Amount**	**Calories**
Coffee, cream, and sugar	1 cup	75
Orange juice	1 cup	110
Soft drinks, juice, punch	12 oz.	140
Diet soft drinks	12 oz.	0
Nonfat milk	1 cup	90
Whole milk	1 cup	160
Milk shake	12 oz.	425
Beer	12 oz.	150
Cocktail	1	150
Mineral water	12 oz.	0

• *Extra fat storage.* If the soft drink calories are *added* to the food calories, the excess will be stored as fat.

• *Uneven blood sugar.* Sugar calories lack fiber and rapidly enter the blood stream, raising blood sugar levels and providing a temporary boost of energy. When the blood sugar level goes up, insulin enters the bloodstream to pull the raised blood sugar back down, and energy levels drop. This sequence promotes the cycle of reaching for another, and yet another, soft drink or other sugary snack.

• *Delayed digestion.* When a sugared drink arrives in a stomach that is processing other food, digestion slows down until the new calories are handled. An occasional drink probably wouldn't make much difference but if it happens several times a day it can prolong digestion and stress the stomach.

• *Acid rebound.* Most beverages, including sodas, increase acid secretion in the stomach. This increase usually occurs after the beverage leaves the stomach, producing a *rebound* effect.

No wonder diet drinks have become so popular!   Is this a good solution?

Diet drinks solve the sugar problems, but that's not the whole story. Most beverages, sugared or not, contain preservatives, flavorings, colorings, and other such chemicals. Some of these substances need to be detoxified and eliminated from the body. They may also irritate sensitive stomach linings.

Most soft drinks, whether diet or not, contain phosphoric acid, a powerful chemical used to etch glass. Americans already consume too much phosphorus, and the body eliminates the extra through the kidneys by combining it with calcium. With today's worries about osteoporosis, the bone-thinning disease, the fact that each phosphorus-containing soft drink may be taking a little calcium with it could be a greater risk than many want to take.

What, then, is the safest way to meet body fluid needs?

Water is the perfect beverage. It has no calories, requires no digestion, does not irritate, and is exactly what the body needs to carry on the life processes. How much should we drink? We should drink enough to keep the urine pale—about six to eight glasses of water daily.

Chapter 18
A Nation of Grazers

Americans spend $10 billion a year on salted snack foods such as potato chips, pork rinds, popcorn and the like. And we spend at least that much more on sweet snacks.

We need snacks, don't we? I read somewhere that it's difficult to get all the nutrients a person needs without snacks.

That bit of wisdom came out of a study done on children. It holds up only when children don't get nourishing, well-balanced meals, or when they aren't hungry enough at mealtime to eat the calories they need.

Most Americans, children or adults, have no real idea what it's like to be hungry. From birth kids are fed almost constantly. The habit carries on through the years. We have become a nation of *grazers*.

But "grazing" is supposed to be a good way to lose weight! You eat a little every hour or so, all day. That way, you don't get hungry, so you don't overeat.

Actually, the calories gained from snacks and beverages can add up to more calories than some people should eat all day!

Suppose, for instance, you have a mid-morning snack of coffee with cream and sugar and a jelly donut.

Add a mid-afternoon snack of a soft drink and a candy bar, plus a late afternoon snack of a cup of coffee with cream and sugar and three cookies.

Top it off in the evening with a typical TV snack: a soft drink, ten potato chips, and five cheese crackers. If this sounds familiar you'd better watch out—all that snacking added approximately 1,500 calories to your day! Now you know why the old saying is still true: *The bigger the snacks, the bigger the slacks.* Many people, as a matter of fact, have gained control of their weight simply by cutting out snacking.

CALORIES FROM SNACKS AND BEVERAGES		
Mid-Morning	Coffee with cream and sugar	75
	Jelly donut	255
Mid-Afternoon	Soft drink	140
	Candy bar	295
Late Afternoon	Coffee with cream and sugar	75
	Cookies (3)	350
TV Snack	Soft drink	140
	Potato chips (10)	125
	Cheese crackers (5)	90
Calories from snacks and beverages		**1,545**

But a lot of people can't get through the day without those *"pick-me-up"* snacks!

That's because they eat refined, fiber-poor, sugar-rich meals, without enough complex carbohydrates (starches) and fiber. A breakfast of sweetened dry cereal and orange juice, for instance (or coffee and donut), is quickly digested. The sugars rush into the bloodstream, push up the blood sugar and provide a temporary high.

But it doesn't hold for long, and when the blood sugar drops, there is a weak, all-gone feeling that cries to be relieved by a beverage or other snack. And the cycle repeats.

A breakfast of whole-grain cooked cereal, whole-wheat bread, and a couple of whole fresh fruits, on the other hand, will furnish plenty of steady energy all morning long. A similarly high-complex carbohydrate, high-fiber lunch will do the same for the afternoon.

Are you saying that we don't need snacks?

The snack habit is just that, *a habit.* With regular, adequate meals there will be much less need for snacks.

What's more, people have fewer digestive problems when they eat simple meals of mostly high-fiber plant foods and then allow their stomachs to rest for awhile. Ideally, meals should be spaced about four to five hours apart.

Any suggestions for a "must have a snack" attack?

Drink a big glass of water. It has no calories and requires no digestion. It passes right through, giving everything a good rinse.

If you must have more, eat a piece of fresh fruit or a handful of raw veggies.

The best way to fight off a *snack attack,* however, is to remember that the calories you save by shunning those snacks will gradually melt off unwanted bulges.

While it may not always be true that *once on the lips, forever on the hips,* there's no more doubting the fact that *the bigger the snacks, the bigger the slacks.*

Chapter 19
Walk Out of Obesity

I n America today, fitness is *in*. Strut your sweat. Lace up your Reeboks. Flaunt your leotards. The majority of Americans, woefully unfit, are feeling out of step.

When I hear that a person has to run 10 miles to work off an ice cream sundae, I feel like—"What's the use!"

There are other choices. You can burn the calories by sleeping for 15 hours or by watching TV for 12 hours. The problem, of course, is that there aren't enough hours in the day to *sleep away* an ice-cream sundae along with your other meals. That's why exercise is so important. It helps your body burn calories faster.

The body is a motor that runs all the time. The rate at which the body motor idles is called its *Basal Metabolic Rate* (BMR). The faster the motor runs, the more fuel is used.

However, when fuel supplies are cut (not enough calories consumed), an inner mechanism turns down the body's idling speed. Available fuel now burns more slowly. This function is life-saving under conditions of starvation, but it defeats the person trying to lose weight.

Can this reaction be prevented?

Activity speeds up the body's metabolic rate. Not only are more calories burned during exercise, but the effect continues for several hours. That's why most people feel more energetic when they exercise. The BMR of the body reflects this. A regular exercise program promotes weight loss by pepping up the metabolism—burning calories faster.

How many calories do I need?

Multiplying your current weight by 10 approximates the daily calories you would need to maintain the status quo if you are bedfast—this is your BMR. Most people use an additional 30 percent of their BMR calories for activity calories. Added together, this figure represents the number of calories you must eat every day to maintain your weight.

If you're fairly sedentary and weigh 150 pounds, for example, your BMR needs would be 1,500 calories, and your activity calories would be 450, for a total of 1,950 calories.

To *lose* weight, you need to reduce this number of calories (eat less) or increase the number of calories used (exercise more). When you develop a negative energy balance, you force your body to burn its reserve fuel, i.e., fat.

Doesn't muscle tissue turn into fat as a person gets older?

Muscle tissue does *not* turn to fat. It is physiologically impossible for this to happen.

When people become less active, however, their muscles shrink and their BMR slows down. Eating habits often are not adjusted to this lessened activity, so as excess calories accumulate, the body stores the fat in numerous places, including the spaces around the muscle fibers.

An important point to understand is that the *muscles burn fat.* When more muscle tissue is present, fat will burn faster and more efficiently.

On the other hand, lack of exercise and overly rigorous dieting will cause the body to *lose* muscle. If this situation persists for a long time, it may become almost impossible to lose further weight.

Is 30 minutes of exercise, three times a week, enough?

Once a person has reached normal weight and a good level of fitness, that may be sufficient. But people who are unfit and people who need to lose weight must aim higher—do an hour a day.

What is the best exercise?

The safest and best exercise is walking; swimming is a close second. People with higher levels of fitness may choose more strenuous exercises.

Start slowly with what you can do. How fast you go isn't the most important thing. What counts is the total distance covered and the duration of the activity. Some people must start with only five minutes at a time several times a day. A person who walks five minutes, carrying 50 pounds of extra weight, will burn more calories than a person carrying only 20 extra pounds who walks the same distance.

If you want to be thin, get in shape. Put your best foot forward, begin to walk your way out of obesity, and keep going for a lifetime!

Chapter 20

Building Caloric Bombs

We often take healthful, nutritious foods and turn them into caloric bombs. It's easy. It's insidious. And we do it without thinking.

Take an apple, for instance. It has vitamins, minerals, fiber, and only 75 to 100 calories. If we ate apples as they come from the tree, we'd have no problem. But we love to douse them with sugar and make applesauce, doubling the calories. Or we squeeze out the juice, removing most of the fiber and concentrating the calories. Even more popular is apple pie, an American special ranked along with motherhood, the flag, and baseball. It's also a nutritional disaster— one slice *a la mode* can easily pack 500 calories..

I could eat a lot of apples for that!

That's the point. You would have to eat five or six apples to reach that caloric level. And you know you wouldn't do that. You'd feel full after two or three.

Or take the potato. By itself the lowly spud is a wonderfully nutritious food. How good is it? Well, a few years ago a scientist tried an experiment. He ate nothing but potatoes for a whole year. Surprisingly, he remained in good heath with plenty of energy.

But look at the way we eat potatoes today. A big 8-oz. potato, by itself, contains about 140 calories. But who eats a plain potato? Here are some of the things we do to dress it up:

		Calories
	with Sour Cream & Butter	**420**
	Hashbrown	**520**
	French Fries	**530**
	Potato Chips	**1,200**
140 calories (8 oz.)	"Pringles"	**1,360**

And that's just the tip of the iceberg. Fresh salads are doused with oily dressings. Most of our fruit goes into juices or pies, or is canned in heavy syrup. Even when we cook fresh vegetables we usually butter them, or add a sauce, which can double and triple the calories. No wonder people have weight problems!

How can we go about reversing this trend?

The solutions are relatively simple. Food preferences, after all, are not inborn, they are learned and cultivated. They can be changed. Substituting a good habit and repeating it over and over with persistence and determination will do the trick.

You can begin by eating more natural foods that have been simply prepared. This includes whole-grain products such as whole-wheat bread, whole-grain cereals, rice, and pasta. It also includes fresh vegetables of all kinds. Tubers like potatoes and yams, and legumes like beans, peas, and lentils are excellent choices.

Indulge yourself with fruit. Whenever possible, eat fresh, whole fruit without added sugar. Peeling and eating an orange, for example, instead of drinking the juice, gives you more food value and fiber and it fills you up with fewer calories.

When food is eaten as grown, it is full of fiber and quite low in calories. By leaving those *caloric bombs* alone, at least most of the time, you can actually eat a larger quantity of food, feel full and satisfied, and still lose weight.

Chapter 21

The Right Weight
Debate

I'm not obese," said one comedian. "I'm just short for my weight!" Whether short or tall, few people are happy about what they weigh.

How can I tell if I'm FIT or FAT?

A person's weight is a highly individual thing but here are some guidelines. By definition, obese means being 20 percent or more above one's ideal weight. A person with an ideal weight of 120 lbs. would be obese at 144 lbs. or more. Overweight, on the other hand, means being 10 percent to 19 percent above one's ideal weight. Our hypothetical person with an ideal weight of 120 lbs. would be overweight at 132 to 143 lbs.

How is your "ideal" weight determined?

Ideal weight can be set in different ways. One way is to look at the records of large life insurance companies who are interested in finding predictors of longevity. They have discovered that certain ideal weight-to-height relationships correlate well with optimum life expectancy. The massive actuarial data of the Metropolitan Life Insurance Company formed the basis of its gender-specific Table of Desirable Weight, based on height and bone size.

IDEAL WEIGHTS FOR ADULTS ACCORDING TO FRAME

Metropolitan Life Insurance Height/Weight Table (1959)+ (Weight in lbs.)*

MEN				WOMEN			
Height (No Shoes)	Small Frame	Medium Frame	Large Frame	Height (No Shoes)	Small Frame	Medium Frame	Large Frame
5'2"	115-123	121-133	129-144	4'10"	96-104	101-113	109-125
4"	121-129	127-139	135-152	5'0"	102-110	107-119	115-131
6"	128-137	134-147	142-161	2"	108-116	113-126	121-138
8"	136-145	142-156	151-170	4"	114-123	120-135	129-146
10"	144-154	150-165	159-179	6"	122-131	128-143	137-154
6'0"	152-162	158-175	168-189	8"	130-140	136-151	145-163
2"	160-171	167-185	178-199	10"	138-148	144-159	153-173
4"	168-179	177-195	187-209				

*Includes one pound for ordinary indoor clothing.
+Many established researchers consider the 1959 table of the Metropolitan Life Insurance Company more consistent with good health than the revised 1983 table with its higher values.

How is bone size calculated?

Although most people have a pretty good idea of their frame size, wrist and sometimes ankle measurements provide a more reliable method. In general, a wrist measurement for women of five and one-quarter inches or less is considered small-boned, between five and one-quarter to six inches is medium, and over six inches is large. For men, anything under six inches is small and anything over seven inches is large.

Is there a simpler way to calculate ideal weight?

Here is a time-honored rule of thumb:

• For men—allow 100 lbs. for five feet of height. For each additional inch, add six pounds. The ideal weight for a man 5' 10" would therefore be 160 lbs.

• For women—also allow 100 lbs. for five feet of height, but add five pounds for each additional inch. For a 5' 5" woman that comes to 125 lbs. Large-boned men and women should add 5 percent to these figures.

Some athletes I know would flunk that test!

That's right, and that's why it's only a rule of thumb. Football players, for instance, have more muscle and greater muscle density than the average person. At the same time they carry very little fat. For this reason, the most accurate way to measure body fat is through hydrostatic (under water) weighing. Fat is buoyant and weighs less under water. This difference allows for calculations of what percentage of a person's body is composed of fat.

One football player consistently weighed in over his maximum allowable weight. He just couldn't lose. Someone finally weighed him under water and found his body fat to be only five percent! (Ideally, a man should have 10 to 15 percent of body weight as fat. For women, 15 percent to 20 percent.)

Where can I get weighed under water?

Look for places that advertise Health Screening tests. Some of them have tanks of water for this purpose. Others use swimming pools. But it's an inconvenient and complicated process.

A simpler, more practical test is the *pinch test.* Trained health professionals use calipers to measure the thickness of skin folds at different places on the body. With the proper tables they can then calculate body fat percentages with fair accuracy.

You can do a simplified pinch test yourself. Reach over to your left side, just below the last rib, and pull the skin and fat away from the underlying muscle. Hold it between your thumb and index finger and squeeze. If the space between your thumb and finger is more than three-fourths of an inch, you're in trouble!

Obesity can be dangerous. Disease and disability follow in its train. Next to quitting smoking, attaining and maintaining an ideal weight is the greatest favor you can do for yourself.

Fail-Safe Formula — Chapter 22

Eat More, Weigh Less

Every second adult in the United States is overweight. Despite 20 years of increasingly sophisticated diets, the average person is now five pounds heavier.

That sounds pretty grim. Is there a brighter side?

Actually, there's a Mr. or Ms. Goodweight inside each one of us—it may just be stuck behind layers of discouragement, bulges of overindulgence, and mounds of misconceptions. We need to locate that special person inside and begin restoring the health, energy, and self-confidence that's been buried far too long.

How do you do that?

By finding a lifestyle that maintains health, increases energy, lowers the risk of disease, reduces food bills, and allows people to eat as much as they want and still lose weight without feeling hungry.

Surely that's an impossible dream!

Not really. Obesity occurs when calories eaten exceed the calories used by the body for physical activity and maintenance of its functions. These leftover calories are stored as fat. By the time 3,500 extra calories have accumulated, one pound of fat will have been deposited.

Adding an extra pat of butter (100 calories) to the daily diet will total up to 10 extra pounds of body fat in one year! On the other hand, omitting dessert (500 fewer calories) for seven days will remove one pound of body fat.

The secret of success lies in finding a way to eat fewer calories instead of eating less food.

That sounds like a contradiction!

Today's world is full of contradictions. Popular magazines and TV screens brim with beautiful, slender people—and with full-color ads of rich, fattening foods. Supermarkets offer 25,000 slickly packaged, calorie-dense products, along with magazines touting the latest quickie diet. Fast food restaurants tempt from nearly every street corner with *takeout* service—but nutrition is what they take out!

Modern food technology, you see, has turned inexpensive, low-calorie, high-volume foods into expensive, high-calorie, low-volume *caloric bombs.* It's now possible to eat a whole meal's worth of calories with only a few bites of food. No wonder people feel hungry and dissatisfied—and overeat!

How does it happen? *Processing* strips seven pounds of sugar beets of their bulk, fiber, and nutrients, producing one pound of *pure sugar.* Sugar and other refined sweeteners now account for about 20 percent of daily calories eaten.

Technology takes 10-14 ears of corn and extracts one tablespoon of corn oil, which, along with its 110 calories, can be swallowed in one gulp! Extracted fats and oils account for another 20 percent of daily calories.

Grains, robbed of fiber and nutrients, can be turned into alcohol accounting for another 9 percent of empty calories many adults consume every day.

Add it up. Almost 50 percent of the modern Western diet consists of processed and concentrated calories devoid of vital nutrients and valuable fiber—a sure-fire formula for overweight.

So how do I go about losing weight?

If you love food but want to lose weight, then—

Eat more . . .

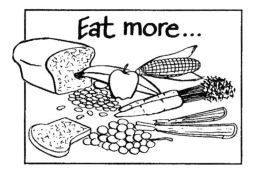

- Fresh and steamed vegetables, but go easy on sauces and salad dressings.

- Whole grains—cooked cereals, brown rice, whole-grain breads, pasta.

- Tubers and other vegetables— potatoes, yams, squash, and all kinds of beans, lentils, and peas.

- Fresh, whole fruits.

These *foods as grown* are filling, nutritious, inexpensive and low in calories.

Eat less . . .

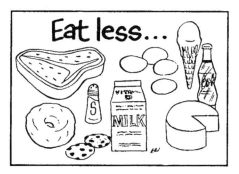

- Refined, processed, and concentrated foods. They are high in calories and price and low in nutrients and fiber.

- Nuts, meats, and rich dairy products. While these foods are nutritious they have little fiber and bulk and are very high in fat and calories. Meats and cheeses, for instance, are 60 percent to 80 percent fat.

What else can I do?

- *Drink plenty of water*—six to eight glasses a day. Try herb teas, mineral water or just plain water. Keep the sodas for special occasions.
- *Walk briskly every day.* Keep at it until you can walk 30 to 60 minutes without fatigue or shortness of breath.
- *Beware of weak moments:*
  - —If one cookie leads to a dozen, don't eat the first one.
  - —Don't buy problem foods. If they are not around you won't be tempted.
  - —If you feel bored, frustrated, or lonely, go for a walk, drink a glass of water, read a book, call a supportive friend. Or, you can *feast* on natural foods like semi-frozen grapes, juicy melons, or crunchy carrot sticks.
- *Tie-in to spiritual resources.* God doesn't make nobodies. He created you for health and prosperity.

It's time to put an end to those unbalanced semi-starvation diets that leave you frustrated, dissatisfied, and craving more to eat. Begin a lifestyle that will recondition your habits toward a lifetime of better health. By avoiding popular trends and choosing the right kinds of foods you can eat more and still lose one to two pounds a week.

UNDERSTANDING FOOD

- Starch
- Sugar
- Bread
- Protein
- Milk
- Meat
- Fat
- Cholesterol
- Fiber
- Salt
- Vitamins

Starch

Chapter 23
A New Superstar

Starchy foods, long shunned as *fattening,* are the new super-stars of the food galaxy. Today's news is that the road to better health is paved with potatoes, pasta, rice, beans, and bread.

What about protein? Everybody needs protein!

Yes, but not so much. For a long time people assumed that because muscles are predominantly protein we needed to eat a lot of it to be strong.

But the body is like a car. Once the car is built, only a few additional parts are needed here and there for maintenance. Similarly, a human adult needs relatively little protein for daily maintenance—around 44 to 61 grams per day. That's about two ounces of pure protein.

What the car does need on a regular basis is good clean gasoline. And carbohydrates are the *gasoline* of the body, the high-octane fuel that keeps it running smoothly.

Isn't fat also a body fuel?

Fat, in general, is stored fuel, carried as baggage. It's the *reserve tank.* If the body runs out of carbohydrate fuel it can dig out the spare stuff. But fat doesn't burn as cleanly as carbohydrates, and it's not as energy efficient.

What are carbohydrates?

Carbohydrates are the sugars and starches in the foods we eat. A lot of people don't understand the relationship between sugars and starches, and the confusion is compounded when terms like *simple carbohydrates* and *complex carbohydrates* are used.

In general, *simple carbohydrates* are the sugars and *complex carbohydrates* are the *starches.* All carbohydrates, both sugars and starches, are broken down by the digestive tract and end up as glucose. The blood absorbs this glucose from the intestines and uses it for energy (fuel). Carbohydrates are almost exclusively found in plant foods—in grains, fruits, and vegetables, and in the many foods made from them, like breads, pastas, pastries, and cereals.

The sugars—*simple carbohydrates*—are digested quickly and, unless fiber is present, they enter the bloodstream as glucose within minutes. This produces a quick rise in blood sugar accompanied by an energy increase. But sugar-flooding often causes the pancreas to overreact, sending out a surge of insulin which not only brings the blood sugar back in line but sometimes drops it too low. The result may be an energy dip, often with a feeling of faintness or shakiness. The usual reaction is to grab a snack or a soda to straighten out the problem.

It works, doesn't it?

A better solution would be to eat an apple. In their natural forms nearly all carbohydrate foods contain liberal amounts of fiber. Although fiber is not generally digested by the body, it absorbs water and forms a soft mass in the intestines which acts to slow down the rate of sugar absorption.

Another solution would be to eat more complex carbohydrates, or starches. Starches are very complex molecules. Larger than sugar molecules, they take longer to digest and thus don't push up the blood sugar level as quickly. The high fiber content of unrefined starchy foods is an additional help in leveling out the rates of digestion and absorption of nutrients.

But aren't starches more fattening than other foods?

Fat is the most fattening food. One gram of fat carries nine calories, while a gram of carbohydrate carries only four calories. Much of the fat we eat goes right into the fat stores of the body.

It's the refining and processing of carbohydrates that causes problems. The volume of the food goes down, while its caloric concentration goes up. That's what makes it so easy to overeat calorically. But when carbohydrates are eaten along with their fiber, the appetite is satisfied with fewer calories.

So what can I eat?

Potatoes and pasta, beans, barley, and rice fill people's stomachs without overloading the system with calories. Add a variety of fruits and vegetables, and it's virtually impossible to eat enough to gain weight.

But top off these healthy foods with butter, gravies, sauces, salad dressings, sour cream, or cheese, and a nutritious, low-calorie food becomes a caloric disaster.

Eating complex carbohydrates as grown, with their full complement of fiber but without those fatty toppings, will not only allow you to eat a greater quantity of food and still lose weight, but will provide you with more consistent energy levels and increased endurance. This kind of eating plan will keep your arteries clean and cut your food bill in half. Where can you find a better bargain than that?

Chapter 24

Chasing the Sugar High

Americans consume an average of 133 pounds of sugars and sweeteners per year for each man, woman, and child. That's nearly three-fourths of a cup a day.

I don't buy that much sugar. Where does it all come from?

Most of the sugar we consume is *hidden* sugar. Here are some of the ways sugar slips into our diets:

- *Soft drinks.* Americans average about 50 gallons of soft drinks per person per year. One 12-oz. soda may contain 12 teaspoons of sugar.

- *Desserts.* A piece of chocolate cake, for instance, contains 15 teaspoons of sugar; a cup of frozen yogurt has 12 teaspoons.

- *Ready-to-eat cereals.* Some, such as *Shredded Wheat* and *Cheerios,* are excellent. But look at cereals like *Fruit Loops* and *Sugar Smacks* with 48 percent and 64 percent of their calories coming from sugar, respectively. This isn't cereal, it's candy!

You'll also find hidden sugar in foods such as canned soups, pot pies, TV dinners, and many brands of peanut butter.

Should I check labels for sugar?

Yes, but realize that sugar may also be *hidden* by giving it a different name. Sucrose, dextrose, lactose, fructose, and maltose, for instance, are all sugars. So are corn syrup, honey, and molasses.

Food	Size Portion	Teaspoons of Sugar
SUGAR CONTENT		
Soft drinks	12 oz.	8-11
Jello, puddings	1 cup	9
Jelly, Jam	2 Tbsp.	10
Pies: apple, berry, cherry, coconut	1 slice	10
Chocolate bar	3 oz.	5
Chocolate mints	4	8
Marshmallow	10	15
Hard candy	4 oz.	20
Raisins	1/2 cup	4
Orange juice (unsweetened)	1 cup	4
Grape juice (commercial)	1 cup	7
Fruit cocktail (commercial)	1 cup	10
Donut (glazed)	1	6
Chocolate chip cookies	4	6
Chocolate eclair	1	7
Angel, pound cake	1 (6 oz.)	9
Gingersnaps	4	12
German chocolate cake	1 (8 oz.)	15
Chocolate milk	1 cup	8
Ice cream, sherbet	1 cup	6-8
Ice cream cone, empty	1 triple	10

Doesn't sugar produce quick energy?

Refined, concentrated sugars enter the bloodstream quickly. Up goes the blood sugar, resulting in a quick energy boost—a sugar high.

But the high is only temporary because it triggers a surge of insulin. Insulin brings down blood sugar levels and in the absence of the moderating effects of fiber sometimes pulls it down too fast and too far.

A falling blood sugar often mimics symptoms of hypoglycemia, producing feelings of weakness, hunger, fatigue, and letdown—the sugar blues. The usual reaction is to reach for another sugary snack, and then another, leading to a sort of *grazing* all day long.

Try eating an apple, a banana, or a bowl of brown rice. The fiber in these foods slows down the absorption of sugar into the bloodstream. The sugar levels won't jump around so much, your energy will stabilize and you'll feel satisfied longer.

Is it true that the body can make sugar out of nearly everything we eat?

Everything but fat. For a long time people thought it didn't really matter what they ate because the body could turn it into whatever it needed. We now know that the way the body processes food, from the time it's eaten until it reaches the bloodstream, makes a great deal of difference.

The body's preferred fuel is glucose, which it makes from sugars and starches (carbohydrates). Although fresh fruits are high in natural sugars they won't strain the body's blood sugar mechanism if they are eaten with their natural fiber.

Starchy foods provide another protection. Starches are broken down more slowly than sugars into the glucose the body needs. Eating starchy foods, especially unrefined starchy foods, along with sugar foods helps stabilize blood sugar levels for extended periods. The ups and downs of the blood sugar curve level off and the insulin response is activated to a lesser degree, if at all.

What are some guidelines for eating sweet foods?

Education and moderation are the secrets.

If you have a sweet tooth, see your dentist . . . well, not really, but a sweet tooth can be reeducated. For instance, fruit is sweet, pleasant to the taste and full of fruit sugars. Practice satisfying your sweet cravings by reaching for a bunch of chilled grapes instead of a donut. Sprinkle slices of strawberries and bananas on your cereal instead of sugar. In time, your tastes will change and you will actually prefer less concentrated sweets.

But this does not mean giving up favorite desserts altogether. *Moderation* is another guideline.

Begin by decreasing the frequency of eating sugared foods. Work from daily (or several times daily) to two or three times a week. When desserts are served less often, you and your family will begin looking forward to them and enjoying them more.

Another aspect of moderation is learning to be satisfied with smaller portions. Big servings and second helpings are just bad habits. You can learn to enjoy one piece of chocolate candy as much as eating the whole box. And you'll feel better! Half of a normal slice of pie or cake, eaten slowly and with pleasure, can be more satisfying than a larger piece bolted down.

Reducing the amount of refined and concentrated sugars in the diet and eating more high-fiber foods, like vegetables, fruits, whole grains, and legumes, will produce the right kind of *sugar highs.* These *highs* will keep you energetic and feeling good all day long.

Bread

Chapter 25

Staff of Life? or Stuff of Lies?

I mitation Bread—Stuff of Lies," is what best-selling author Dr. David Rubin calls today's white bread. "It's a bizarre combination of the least nutritious part of the wheat grain and a number of artificial chemicals, which can be harmful."

What's wrong with white bread?

Basically, what's wrong is what the milling process does to wheat. A grain of wheat is made up of an outer covering (bran), an embryo (wheat germ) and the endosperm.

The bran contains most of the fiber, generous amounts of vitamins and minerals and a bit of protein.

The germ is a rich source of B and E vitamins, several minerals, and fiber.

The endosperm, which makes up roughly four-fifths of the whole wheat kernel, contains protein (gluten) and starch. It is the only part used in making white flour. Ironically, the nutritious bran and wheat germ, which are removed during the milling process, are sold for animal feed.

The food industry further compounds the nutritional problems by using several artificial chemicals, such as:

BRAN

ENDOSPERM

BRAN

EMBRYO, OR WHEAT GERM

- Propylene glycol (antifreeze) to keep bread white.
- Diacetyltartaric acid (an emulsifier) to save on shortening.
- Calcium sulfate (plaster of Paris) to make it easier to knead large batches of dough.

Should we avoid eating white bread?

No bread is all bad. Even the white, fluffy stuff is a high starch and low-fat food. It's just that some breads are much better than others.

Take fiber, for instance. A slice of white bread contains one-quarter gram of fiber, while a slice of 100 percent whole wheat bread contains two grams, and some multi-grain breads contain as much as three and one-half grams of fiber per slice. This means you'd need to eat eight or more slices of white bread to get the fiber of one slice of whole-grain bread.

What about enriched flour and enriched bread?

During the milling of wheat at least 24 known minerals and vitamins are largely removed. When nutritional deficiency diseases emerged around the turn of the century, as a result of commercial milling, the industry started an enrichment program. Four of the nutrients were restored—thiamine, riboflavin, niacin, and iron. However, in most cases, nothing has been done about the other lost nutrients.

% LOSS OF NUTRIENTS WHEN REFINING WHEAT

Thiamine (B_1)	86%	Calcium	50%
Riboflavin (B_2)	70%	Phosphorus	78%
Niacin (B_3)	80%	Copper	75%
Iron	84%	Magnesium	72%
Pyridoxine (B_6)	60%	Manganese	71%
Folic Acid	70%	Zinc	71%
Pantothenic Acid	54%	Chromium	87%
Biotin	90%	Fiber	68%

What kind of bread is the most healthful?

Truly healthful bread contains ground up whole grains, with the bran, wheat germ, and endosperm present. Such breads have double, triple, and in some cases quadruple nutrient value when compared with their refined counterparts.

When combined with fresh fruit, cereals, vegetables, potatoes, and beans, bread makes interesting and satisfying meals and helps maintain good energy levels for long periods.

Look for the substantial-feeling loaves that aren't full of air. Look for 100 percent whole wheat, stone ground if possible. Sprouted-wheat breads are also excellent.

Find a reliable bakery. Better yet, make your own bread.

Whole-wheat flour seems to attract weevils!

Whole-grain flours have a healthy balance of starch, protein, natural fats, and fiber besides being loaded with vitamins and minerals. The bugs seem to know this. White flour, on the other hand, is such a nutritional minus that they usually won't touch it.

Store whole-grain flours in your refrigerator or freezer. Or buy the grains whole and grind them up into flour just before using.

Isn't bread, even whole-wheat bread, fattening?

It isn't the bread that's fattening but what's done to it. A slice of whole-wheat bread has 70 calories—no more than an apple. If slathered with peanut butter and jam, the slice can pack close to 300 calories. It's not the raw materials but the overhead that can turn a low-calorie, nutritious, healthful slice of good bread into a caloric disaster.

Bread has traditionally been the backbone of human nutrition. Restoring good bread to its rightful place is a big step toward better health. Next time you shop for bread go for the real *Staff of Life.*

"Wherefore do you spend money for that which is not bread? and your labor for that which satisfieth not? hearken diligently unto me, and eat that which is good."
—Isaiah 55:2

Chapter 26

Exploding the Myth

A sk almost any 14-year-old boy whether he would rather grow bigger faster, or live longer, and he would probably choose the former.

Is that a relevant question?

Yes, because in the 1930s studies on laboratory animals began to turn up evidence that high protein diets accelerated growth rate and maturation, but shortened life span.

In animals, maybe. But everyone knows that humans need plenty of protein!

Back in 1880 a German scientist, Dr. Liebig, determined that muscles were made of protein. Dr. Karl Voit, watching coal miners in Munich, calculated that these strong, muscular men ate around 120 grams of protein a day and announced that this was the ideal amount to eat. Getting enough protein grew to be an obsession, a myth that persists to this day.

A myth? Are you saying we don't need protein?

Modern scientific studies show that adults actually need only about 20 to 30 grams of protein a day. The human body very efficiently harvests and recycles its own protein. The only protein losses that need to be replaced are those that the body cannot retrieve, such as hair, finger and toe nails, and skin.

So we need only 20-30 grams of protein a day?

Remember that the National Academy of Sciences sets the RDA (Recommended Daily Allowance) for vitamins, minerals, and certain foods by determining how much the body needs each day, then doubling that amount. Thus the RDA for protein has been set at 0.35 grams per pound of body weight. That works out to 60 grams for a 170-lb. man and 42 grams for a 120-lb. woman. Even though this is more than enough, the average Westerner continues to eat between 100 to 120 grams of protein a day.

What is the problem with that?

• Most of the protein eaten by Westerners comes from animal sources and is loaded with cholesterol and saturated fat. Because fat is well hidden, many people don't realize that meats and dairy products average from 50 percent to 85 percent of their calories as fat calories. Excess fat and cholesterol, and especially *saturated* fat, are known for their atherosclerosis-promoting effects, which lead to narrowing, hardening, and increase of plaque in vital oxygen-carrying arteries. This process ACCELERATES AGING AND SHORTENS LIFE.

• From 1850 to 1990 the average age of sexual maturity for teenage girls declined from 17.5 years to 11.9 years.

• A high protein diet is not conducive to endurance. Athletes now load up with carbohydrates rather than protein.

• Excess protein places added burdens on the kidneys. Kidney disease is increasingly common in Western culture.

• High protein diets are being associated with osteoporosis. The processing of excess protein by the kidneys requires calcium, much of which comes directly from bone stores.

Don't children need extra protein?

Yes, they do, especially during periods of rapid growth. The RDA of 0.35 grams per pound of body weight works out to 17.5 grams

PROTEIN CONTENT IN FOOD PRODUCTS			
U.S. Diet	**Grams**	**Optimal Diet**	**Grams**
3-Egg Ham and Cheese Omelet	46	Cooked Cereal	9
Hashbrown Potatoes	3	with Milk and ½ Banana	11
Toast (2) with Butter, Jelly	5	Toast (2) with ½ Banana	4
Orange Juice	1	Fruit (Orange)	1
Breakfast Total	**55**	**Breakfast Total**	**25**
		Pita Bread (3) stuffed with	
Big Mac	26	Tomatoes, Sprouts, Cucumbers	8
French Fries	3	Three Bean Salad	10
Milk Shake	11	Split Pea Soup with Barley	12
Lunch Total	**40**	**Lunch Total**	**30**
Fried Chicken (basket)	40	Spaghetti with Tomato Sauce	10
Mixed Salad, Dressing	4	Tossed Salad	4
Baked Potato, Sour Cream	8	Broccoli Flowerets	5
Peas	5	Bread (2) with Garbanzo Spread	10
Milk	10	Baked Apple with Walnuts	1
Dinner Total	**67**	**Dinner Total**	**30**
Total Grams of Protein	162	Total Grams of Protein	85

of protein a day for a 50-lb. child—a little over half an ounce. Since children in Western cultures eat the same excessively high protein diets that adults do, they are not likely to experience protein deficiencies when food supplies are adequate.

The problem may well be on the other side of the question. Accumulating evidence suggests that children eating high-fat and protein diets tend to grow bigger and to develop faster. Are they paying the price of a shortened life?

What about the amino acid arguments?

Proteins are made of some 20 amino acids. While the body can manufacture twelve of these building blocks, eight amino acids have been demonstrated to be essential for adults. They have to be provided by the diet. People used to believe that they had to eat meat and dairy products in order to supply these "essential" amino acids. The fact that these foods are high in fat and cholesterol, lack fiber, and have detrimental effects on health was, for many years, overlooked or considered irrelevant.

Now we know that these amino acids are easily available from a random selection of plant foods. This is shown in dietary patterns around the world. The staple food in Caribbean countries is black beans and rice. The amino acids missing in rice are found in the beans, and vice versa. The same is true for the corn tortillas and pinto beans of the Mexicans, and the rice and soy beans relied upon by the Chinese.

The Western world is taking a fresh look at plant foods. They are low in fat, high in fiber, free of cholesterol, and have plenty of protein. The protein content of many vegetables exceeds 20 percent of total calories, while whole grains average about 12 percent and most seeds and legumes around 20-30 percent.

Progressive nutritionists advise getting 10 percent of daily calories as protein. Even on a total vegetarian diet, getting this much protein is obviously no problem. In fact, when enough calories are available from a variety of unrefined plant foods, it's virtually impossible to create a protein deficiency.

It's time to bury the myth and catch up with the times. Decreasing the amount of protein you eat to RDA levels is a good place to start. With protein, as with much else in life, too much of a good thing is a bad thing.

Milk

Chapter 27

Who Needs It?

Milk is the perfect food—for babies; mother's milk, that is. There are about 4,300 species of mammals on earth, and each mammal's milk is precisely designed and balanced for its own young.

Are you saying that cow's milk shouldn't be given to human babies?

It's looking more and more that way. The American College of Pediatrics no longer recommends animal milk for children under one year of age. Reasons? Iron absorption problems, allergies, colic, eczema, nasal and bronchial conjestion.

What about the rest of us? Isn't milk a healthful food?

For years we've been led to believe that milk is indispensable for sound health. However, the average Westerner eats too much fat, too much cholesterol, too much protein and not enough fiber. While milk, when calculated in percent of calories, is 50 percent fat (much of it saturated) and 20 percent protein. It contains cholesterol and has no dietary fiber. Drinking milk puts added burdens on an already overloaded metabolic system.

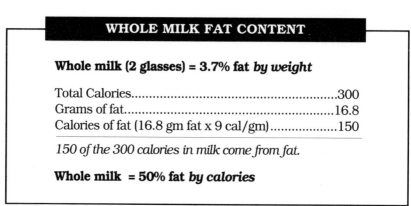

How about lowfat milk? Doesn't that solve most of the problems?

Lowfat milk is an improvement over whole milk, but not as great as it seems. The 2 percent fat in lowfat milk is calculated from the weight of the milk, not from its calories. By weight, this milk is 87 percent water and 2 percent fat. By calories, lowfat milk is a 30 percent fat food.

Nonfat milk (skim milk) is the best choice for those who wish to drink milk. It has no fat and only a trace of cholesterol yet retains its other nutrients.

How about calcium? Isn't milk famous for its calcium content?

It's true that milk is high in calcium, but before choosing to drink milk, people need to balance its calcium advantage against its problems. Here are a few:

• The incidence of coronary heart disease in North America is much higher than in non-milk-drinking cultures. Whole milk, with its saturated fat and cholesterol, contributes to heart disease.

• Cultures with the highest milk consumption have the highest rates of osteoporosis, a disease rarely found in non-milk-drinking countries. Instead of protecting against osteoporosis, a high dairy consumption may actually contribute to the bone-thinning process.

This happens because metabolizing excess protein can leach calcium out of the bones.

• Each animal's milk is designed to fit the growth rates of its own young. Human babies develop very slowly, and the composition of human milk reflects that difference. Animal milks may contribute to the earlier maturation noted in many of today's children.

• After weaning, humans have a high percentage of lactose intolerance (inability to properly digest milk sugar) evidenced by excessive gas, cramps, and diarrhea. Roughly 75 percent of the world's population show some degree of this problem.

• Milk is the most common cause of food allergies. More than 100 antigens (perpetuators of allergies) may be released by the normal digestion of cow's milk. Many people with diseases such as asthma, rheumatoid arthritis, and hay fever, do better when they stop drinking milk.

• Most Westerners eat too much protein, and milk is a high protein food.

• Milk is a common cause of constipation.

• Milk can also transmit disease, unless it is sterilized (as opposed to pasteurized). It frequently contains residues of antibiotics, hormones, pesticides, and other drugs that were added to the cow's feed.

Many concerned people are choosing other sources of calcium such as grains, legumes, vegetable greens, and if needed, supplements.

Are you implying that adult humans don't need milk?

Many people live their whole lives in good health without drinking milk or using other dairy products. If used, milk should be consumed—preferably in nonfat form—in small quantities, such as in cooking, or on breakfast cereal.

Consider this: Outside of zoos, no mammal consumes the milk of another species, and once weaned, no mammal again consumes milk. Humans are the exception.

Every creature's milk is a health food only for its own offspring.

Chapter 28

Looking for the Real Food

Real Food! In fact, Real Food for Real People! What an attractive thought! What an exciting promise!

Real food? What does that mean?

In the commercials, *Real Food* turned out to be beef, and attractive celebrities lauded its virtues. An authoritative voice explained that three ounces of the new, leaner cuts of beef contained no more cholesterol than three ounces of chicken.

What the voice didn't tell you was that lean beef, while comparable to chicken in cholesterol content, contains three to six times more dangerous, cholesterol-raising saturated fat. Besides, who eats 3-oz. portions? The average hamburger weighs close to five ounces and an average-size steak weighs about six ounces.

But isn't meat an important source of protein?

Meat is a nutritious source of protein but it carries along a number of problems:

For one thing, most people overestimate their protein needs. The Recommended Daily Allowance (RDA) for protein is a generously adequate 44-61 grams, yet most Westerners consume two to three times this much. And much of the excess is derived from animal foods.

Following World War II, for example, Americans averaged around 50 pounds of meat, per person/per year. Today we more than double that figure for beef alone. And the consumption of poultry and fish is skyrocketing. Yet we've known for years that excessive amounts of protein are toxic to the kidneys.

An even bigger problem is the hefty doses of fat (mostly saturated) and cholesterol that a serving of meat carries. Scientific research has overwhelmingly implicated a *rich diet* as the major culprit in today's diseases. And the rich foods that are doing us in are mostly animal products, such as meat, eggs, and dairy products.

The trouble is, while the human body is able to nourish itself on animal foods, it lacks the special protection against large amounts of fat and cholesterol that carnivorous animals have. In humans, excessive fat and cholesterol stack up in the bloodstream and begin attaching to the linings of blood vessels. Gradually, over time, arteries thicken and narrow, and plaque forms.

As blood supplies to vital organs diminish or are cut off, the stage is set for many of today's killer diseases, such as heart disease, hypertension, stroke, diabetes, and several types of cancer.

Are you suggesting that a meatless lifestyle is better?

There are millions of people around the world getting along just fine on plant protein diets. Consider some of the advantages:

Decreased risk of disease: Vegetarian populations are remarkably free of the killer diseases that are ravishing Westernized countries.

Healthier longevity: Statistically, vegetarians are thinner, healthier, and live longer than the average person.

Increased food safety:

- As soon as an animal dies, enzymes are released which begin the process of decay. Proper preservation of meat is a continuing challenge.
- Animals ingest and store chemicals in their bodies from the fertilizers and pesticides used on their food.
- Inspectors must check carcasses rapidly, making careful examinations difficult.
- Random sampling reveals that meat frequently contains residues of growth hormones and antibiotics. Although there are laws controlling this, they are difficult to enforce.
- Today most food animals are raised on feedlots or contained in cages, with practically no exercise. The meat from these animals may contain up to twice as much fat as the meat from range-fed and free farm animals.

Environmental protection: Twenty-five gallons of water will produce one pound of wheat, whereas 2,500 gallons are needed to produce one pound of beef.

Increased world food supplies: Eighty percent to 90 percent of the grain grown in the U.S.A. is fed to animals. If Americans would reduce their meat consumption by 50 percent, the land, water, grain, and soybeans saved would feed the entire developing world.

What's happened to natural food? Isn't that considered real food anymore?

Promoters love to extol the virtues of natural foods. Originally, the term meant foods from whole plants. Through years of careless use, however, its meaning has broadened until today it is used to refer to almost anything that contains at least one healthful ingredient.

The evidence against meat and other animal products is stacking up as nutritional research confirms that a diet built around whole plant food is not only adequate, but superior.

However, promoting health and preventing disease through

diet and lifestyle does not always advance profit margins. For this reason we will continue to be bombarded by expensive ads seducing us to buy products with inadequate attention to health consequences.

Humans don't have the instinct to kill. We are more apt to salivate over a bunch of cold grapes than a piece of raw meat. It's comforting to know that a diet of fruit, vegetables, legumes, and grains is perfectly suited to our needs—anatomically and physiologically as well as instinctively.

The wise among us will not look to the slaughterhouses for *real food*. The wise among us will find *real food* in the gardens and farms of our land.

Fat

Chapter 29

Why All the Fuss?

An insidious villain is at work in our country quietly disabling and killing more Americans each year than all the wars in this century. *That villain is the fat in our food!*

Are you saying that eating fat can kill us?

The excess fat in food is being singled out as the most damaging component of the Western diet. That deadly duo—the high-fat, low-fiber diet—is now linked to such diverse problems as coronary artery (heart) disease, gallstones, appendicitis, cancers of the colon, breast, and prostate, strokes, constipation, diverticulitis, and gout, to name a few. And the list continues to grow.

Don't we need fat to be healthy?

Fat is a vital part of every living cell. Fat is also the body's back-up fuel system. We could not be optimally healthy without fat in our diets.

Problems occur because most of us eat too much fat, often in forms the body cannot easily handle. We understand that a car runs best with its specified fuel. We might get a car to run on kerosene, but it would be disastrous to its engine. Improper fuel damages the body motor also, though it's not as readily seen because a healthy body has great reserves. Up to 90 percent of the liver and kidneys can be destroyed before the organs go into failure. By the time the first anginal pain or heart attack is experienced, the diameter of coronary arteries in important locations may already be reduced by 80 percent to 90 percent.

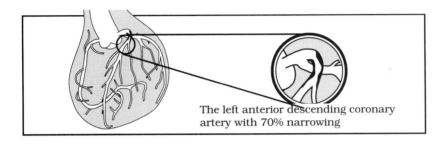

The left anterior descending coronary artery with 70% narrowing

How does fat damage the body?

An excessive amount of fat in the diet sets up conditions for the development of atherosclerosis—a hardening and narrowing of vital arteries that supply food and oxygen to the body. Excess fat makes the blood thick and sticky, slowing circulation and causing

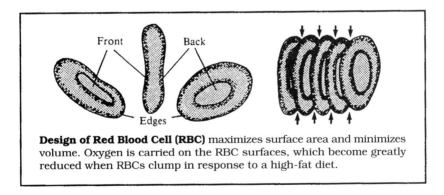

Design of Red Blood Cell (RBC) maximizes surface area and minimizes volume. Oxygen is carried on the RBC surfaces, which become greatly reduced when RBCs clump in response to a high-fat diet.

red blood cells to adhere to each other in bunches. These clumped blood cells cannot carry their full load of oxygen, and they are unable to navigate tiny capillaries. Deprived of oxygen and nutrients, body cells become susceptible to injury, disease, and death.

Most high fat foods are loaded with cholesterol which injures the linings of arteries. The body responds by sealing off these damaged spots with extra cells. In the presence of excess fat and cholesterol more and more *band-aids* are added, one on top of the other, until plaques are formed. When plaques grow large enough to narrow and obstruct coronary arteries, heart attacks occur. When it happens in arteries feeding the brain, a stroke takes place.

Some of the by-products of fat digestion appear to be involved in the promotion of certain cancers. These substances often cause irritation and inflammation of bowel walls, and may be a factor in colitis and colon cancer. When adequate fiber is present, however, feces move along quickly, leaving less time for toxic carcinogens to act on bowel walls.

On another front, exess fat in the bloodstream is one of the factors that depresses immune cell production.

WHERE IS THE FAT?		
Foods	**% Fat Calories**	**Total Calories Per Cup (8 oz.)**
Visible Fats		
Butter, Margarine, Shortening, Lard	98-100%	1650-1900
Invisible Fats		
Peanut Butter	80%	1500
Nuts	75-92%	800
Pork, Beef	65-80%	500-800
Double Beef Whopper (Burger King)	59%	970
Whole Milk	50%	160
Ice Cream	70-80%	350
Processed Cheese	60-85%	450
Cream Cheese	90%	850

High-fat diets have been shown to impair the efficiency of the body's insulin mechanism, which may lead to diabetes. The amount of saturated fat in the diet also powerfully affects blood cholesterol levels.

What can we do to protect ourselves?

It's crucial that we cut down on the fat in our diets. Butter, margarine, shortening, cooking and salad oils are nearly 100 percent fat. Meats, cheeses, eggs, and whole milk average 50 percent to 80 percent of calories as fat.

Furthermore, we need a big increase in fiber intake. Fruits, vegetables, whole grains, and legumes are gaining in popularity. Because these plant foods are high in fiber, low in fat and free of cholesterol, they are the ideal way to go.

The Western diet, bloated with fat, is slowly killing us. We know now that the situation can be turned around by replacing most of the fat calories we eat with unrefined plant foods.

A diet balanced in this manner will prevent many Western-type diseases and help reverse coronary heart disease and most adult diabetes. And there is more. You will enjoy better health and feel more energetic. You can also eat a higher volume of food and lose weight too!

Chapter 30
Cholesterol Countdown

What can turn a normal, needed, healthful substance into a dangerous killer? How can something that makes sex hormones, helps build strong bones, and balances the body's stress response also choke off oxygen and damage vital organs and tissues?

Cholesterol is both hero and villain. While we cannot live without it, in excessive amounts it can kill us.

The blood cholesterol level is the single most important factor in determining a person's risk for heart disease, the nation's number one killer. A person with a blood cholesterol level of 260 mg% (6.8 mmol/L) is four times more likely to have a fatal heart attack than is a person with a cholesterol of less than 200 mg% (5.1 mmol/L).

Doesn't heredity determine cholesterol level?

Very few people have genetic cholesterol disorders. Most cholesterol levels are determined by dietary factors. Depending on what people eat, cholesterol levels can go up or down substantially within a few weeks.

How does high cholesterol cause heart attacks?

It does it by gradually plugging up the vital arteries that nourish the heart through a process called atherosclerosis.

Most heart attacks are related to plaques which are made up mostly of cholesterol and fat. Plaques are like tire patches. They are the body's response to damaged areas in arterial walls. In response to continuing irritation over the years, the plaque slowly enlarges while endeavoring to *protect* the area. But in doing so it also chokes off the blood flow and may eventually obstruct the artery completely.

When blood cholesterol levels are under 160 mg% (4.1 mmol/L), initial arterial damage usually heals quickly and the scars shrink. But when cholesterol levels edge past 200 (5.1 mmol/L), LDL-cholesterol somehow attaches itself with greater ease to the vessel walls causing thickening, stiffening, narrowing, and plaque formation.

Massive studies of world populations have documented the fact that blood cholesterol levels are the most dependable predictor of arterial obstructions due to plaque formation. Research on migrant groups of people confirms that this is not so much a disease of genetics as it is of lifestyle. When people who have been protected by a simple diet move into a Westernized culture with its dietary excesses, their blood cholesterol levels go up and they soon begin developing the same arterial diseases as Westerners.

But doesn't the body need cholesterol?

Yes, but we don't have to eat it. The liver manufactures all the cholesterol the body needs. But most Westerners eat an additional 400-500 mg of cholesterol a day. It's this extra cholesterol that causes the trouble.

What foods contain cholesterol?

Cholesterol is found *only* in animal foods. Plant foods do not contain cholesterol. It's as simple as that (see table on the next page).

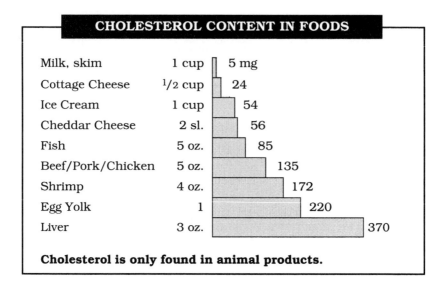

CHOLESTEROL CONTENT IN FOODS

Food	Amount	Cholesterol
Milk, skim	1 cup	5 mg
Cottage Cheese	1/2 cup	24
Ice Cream	1 cup	54
Cheddar Cheese	2 sl.	56
Fish	5 oz.	85
Beef/Pork/Chicken	5 oz.	135
Shrimp	4 oz.	172
Egg Yolk	1	220
Liver	3 oz.	370

Cholesterol is only found in animal products.

I've heard that coconut and palm oils raise cholesterol levels.

Yes, that's true. Even though these tropical fats do not contain cholesterol, they are high in saturated fats. Saturated fats can substantially raise cholesterol levels all by themselves. They do this by stimulating the liver's cholesterol output.

Saturated fats are mostly found in animal foods like meat, eggs, and dairy products and most are solid at room temperature.

What is a safe blood cholesterol level?

Many heart researchers suggest that cholesterol levels under 160 mg% (4.1 mmol/L) will protect people from atherosclerosis.

What are some practical ways to lower cholesterol?

- *Eat less cholesterol.* Reduce the amount of cholesterol eaten to under 100 mg a day. This means markedly reducing meat, especially organ meats, and sausages, egg yolks and most dairy products.
- *Eat less saturated fat.* As mentioned, these fats are found

mostly in animal products but they also occur in palm and coconut oil, shortening, and some margarines.

- *Lose excess weight.* Cutting down on highly refined empty calorie foods, such as visible fats and oils, sugar and alcohol, helps here.
- *Eat more fiber.* High fiber foods help lower blood cholesterol. Eat plenty of unrefined starches, fresh fruits, and vegetables, whole grains, beans, potatoes, and yams.
- *Exercise.* Walk daily. Regular exercise helps reduce blood cholesterol levels and aids weight control.
- *Medications.* Check with your physician for advice about whether you need cholesterol-lowering medications.

Remember, blood cholesterol is directly affected by the richness of the diet. A diet *very low* in fat (less than 15 percent of calories) and high in fiber has been shown to lower most blood cholesterol levels by 20 percent to 35 percent in less than four weeks.

If you don't know what your blood cholesterol level is, don't walk, run to the nearest checkpoint. If the result is over 160 mg% (4.1 mmol/L), it's time to get serious!

Chapter 31

Are Juicers the Answer?

The commercials are attractive; the live demonstrations are astounding. Piles of magnificent-looking fresh produce are fed into a little machine—and presto—beautiful juice!

Across the country busy people, accustomed to technological wonders and dedicated to health improvement, are welcoming yet another exciting shortcut to the good life: fruit and vegetable juicers.

Are these juicers as good as they claim?

Yes and no. Yes, they produce a nutritious drink, but, no, most do not live up to the health claims that are all too often made for them.

While juice machines deliver a product that is fairly rich in nutrients, most do so at the expense of valuable food fiber. Ten pounds of fresh produce may yield two quarts of delicious juice. But nearly all the precious *fiber,* that the body so badly needs, is in the five or six pounds of *pulp* that go down the garbage disposal.

The process is reminiscent of the mills of 100 years ago that began removing bran and germ (fiber and nutrients) from grains, leaving low-fiber, nutrient-poor residues like white flour and white rice. Unfortunately these foods are still the mainstay of much of the current world population.

Just what is fiber?

Fiber is the framework of plants. Because it passes through the body without being absorbed by the blood, it was long thought to be of no value. Removing it increased the caloric value of food and the efficiency and speed with which it was absorbed into the bloodstream. It also prolonged its shelf life.

The many kinds of fiber fall into two basic groups—those that dissolve in water (soluble fiber) and those that don't (insoluble fiber).

What does fiber do?

Fiber is like a general, controlling many different body processes.

• Insoluble fiber absorbs and holds water—from four to six times its own volume—creating soft, spongy masses in the stomach and intestines. The result? A sense of fullness occurs much sooner than with low-fiber foods, helping to protect against overeating and aiding in weight control.

• The fiber masses, acting like soaked-up sponges, fill the intestines more completely and stimulate them to lively activity. Instead of idling for several days in the gastrointestinal tract in compacted lumps, as low-fiber foods do, the spongy masses pass along much more quickly and are evacuated in 24 to 36 hours.

This action cures most constipation and significantly relieves problems with hemorrhoids and diverticular disease.

• Because of the shorter transit time, there is less putrefaction (decomposition of organic material) in the intestines. There is less time for carcinogens and other harmful end-products to irritate the bowel walls. The fiber also provides insulation against damaging food residues. These fiber-related actions may explain the lower colon cancer rates among people with higher fiber intakes.

• Fiber also slows down the rate at which nutrients enter the bloodstream. This helps smooth out the ups and downs of blood sugar levels and provides more consistent energy throughout the day. A stabilized blood sugar relieves most hypoglycemia (low blood sugar) and aids in the control of diabetes (high blood sugar).

• Soluble fiber, on the other hand, helps lower blood cholesterol levels. It does this by attaching to cholesterol by-products and pulling them out of the intestines before the body can reabsorb them.

Where do you find this seeming miracle worker?

Fiber is abundant in all unrefined plant foods. Eating a variety of fruits, whole grains, vegetables, and legumes (beans, lentils, peas) assures a plentiful supply of the many varieties of fiber the body needs.

For people who find it hard to chew fresh food, there are juice machines available which retain food fiber. The product is thick, like pudding, but can be diluted like ordinary juice concentrate.

What about meat and dairy products?

Most people are surprised to learn that animal foods do not contain any fiber. And since meat, poultry, fish, eggs, and dairy products make up more than 30 percent of the calories of the typical Western diet, and much of the rest comes from sugars and other refined foods, the result is that most Westerners get only about one-third of the fiber they need each day.

What about adding wheat bran to food?

Adding wheat bran can be helpful to sedentary people on limited diets. But most people don't need fiber pills, extracted brans, and other expensive supplements. It would take a whole bottle of fiber pills to supply the fiber contained in a bowl of whole-grain cereal topped with strawberries. Fiber is not something you can sprinkle on a plate of steak and eggs and make it OK.

Fiber-poor foods are hazardous to your health. Don't be misled by gimmicks that tamper with the balance of natural foods.

Focus on whole-grain cereals and breads, fresh fruit and vegetables, and plenty of beans and other legumes. This is the healthiest, safest, cheapest, and best way to get the fiber you need.

Chapter 32

Is Salt Losing Favor?

Americans and most other Westernized people eat up to 20 times more salt than they need. And they pay for it with high blood pressure, heart failure, and other problems related to fluid retention.

Don't we need salt?

Salt contains two minerals, sodium and chloride. Sodium is the important one; every cell contains sodium, as do all body fluids. We couldn't live without it. But while it is essential for body metabolism, sodium can also cause trouble.

How does salt raise blood pressure?

Excess sodium can stay in body tissues and hold extra water. This causes swelling which raises the blood pressure, which in turn increases stress on the heart. Every third American adult now has an elevated blood pressure. Over age 65, the figures rise to 70 percent.

The average salt intake in Japan is even higher than in the U.S.A. and so is the prevalence of hypertension. Stroke, a complication of hypertension, is the leading cause of death in Japan.

In other societies, such as those in rural Uganda or the Amazon basin, where salt intake is very low, hypertension is virtually unknown even in advanced age. Dr. Lot Page, a respected researcher, states categorically, "Without exception, low-blood-pressure societies are low-salt societies. Conversely, mass hypertension follows mass salt consumption."

Is this true for everyone?

Not everyone is salt sensitive. Some people can eat all they want without ill effects. As many as one-half of Americans have some vulnerability to salt, however, and there is no satisfactory test for identifying them.

Salt-sensitive people retain sodium, which causes edema (swelling). Many people carry five to seven extra pounds of water weight because of excess salt in their bodies. Decreasing salt intake allows the body to shed the excess water.

Some 30 million Americans with mild essential hypertension could normalize their blood pressures by cutting their salt intake to one teaspoon (five grams) a day.

Besides weight and blood pressure control, such a low-salt diet favorably affects P.M.S. (premenstrual syndrome), certain headaches, and some depressions. And it reduces the water logging in chronic heart failure.

What about water pills?

Water pills successfully lower blood pressure by eliminating extra water. But recent research reveals that diuretics may actually contribute to heart disease by increasing cholesterol levels 5 percent to 10 percent. Over time, these drugs may also damage the kidneys, promote gout, and accelerate diabetes. Eliminating extra water by natural means is the safer way to go.

Don't people who take diuretics for high blood pressure have to take them for life?

That was yesterday's news. The word today is that up to 85 percent of hypertensives can be eased off water pills in response to a low-salt, low-fat diet combined with weight loss and daily walking.

But I can't stand saltless food!

Salt preferences are not inborn. *Saltiness* is a learned habit, and eating salty foods fuels the craving. Salt masks natural flavors. Shake the habit by seasoning with herbs and spices. Give yourself three weeks. After that, even so-called normal foods will begin to taste salty. For the diehards, use salt substitutes.

What are some high-sodium foods to avoid?

Watch out for baking soda, baking powder, MSG (mono-sodium glutamate), salty snacks, and anything pickled. Eat less processed foods (chocolate pudding has more sodium than potato chips), baked goods, meats, dairy products, and presweetened cereals. Especially shun canned vegetables unless labeled "no salt added." One tablespoon of canned peas contains as much sodium as five pounds of fresh peas!

How much salt is safe to eat?

FOOD PROCESSING — HIDDEN SALT

FOOD Natural State	SALT (mg)	FOOD Commercial, Processed	SALT (mg)
Apple (1 fresh)	5	Apple Pie (1 slice)	500
White Beans (1 cup)	12	Chili & Beans (1 cup)	3,000
Rice, Brown (1 cup)	12	Minute Rice (1 cup)	1,000
Wheat Flakes (2 oz.)	20	Wheaties (2 oz.)	1,850
Potato (1 fresh, 5 oz.)	20	Potato Chips (5-oz. bag)	3,500
Tomato (1 fresh)	35	Tomato Sauce (1/2 cup)	1,950
		Tomato Soup (1 cup)	2,200
Beef, lean	140	Corned Beef	2,360
Milk (1 cup)	300	Cheese, Amer. (2 slices)	2,050
Chicken (8 oz.)	300	Kentucky Fried Chicken (3-piece dinner)	5,600

Most people are genuinely amazed at how little sodium (salt) the body actually needs in a day—an average of about half a gram or 1/10th *teaspoon,* since some sodium occurs naturally in food.

However, this is too drastic a change for most of us. Concentrate on cutting down. Instead of 10 to 20 grams, limit yourself to one teaspoon (5 grams) of salt a day. This is a reasonably safe limit for most people.

Here are some ideas to help you decrease the salt in your diet:

- Eat lots of fresh, raw foods, both fruits and vegetables. They need no added salt. They also increase potassium stores, which help lower blood pressure.
- Look for unsalted snacks (if you need them).
- Undercook vegetables and eat them a bit crispy. They will require less salt.
- Toast (dextrinize) bread and cereals for added flavor.
- Learn to flavor foods with lemon juice, fresh herbs, parsley, tarragon, garlic, and onions, instead of with salt.
- Take advantage of the excellent salt-free gourmet cookbooks available on the market today.

The average American consumes 15 pounds of salt a year. Reducing this to four pounds would be a major step toward better health.

SALT "BOMBS"		
Condiment	**Amount**	**Salt (mg)**
Ketchup	3 tsp	1,100
Italian Dressing	3 tsp	2,500
Soy Sauce	1 tsp	2,500
Dill Pickle	1 large	3,000
Garlic Salt	1 tsp	4,500
Salt	1 tsp	5,000

Megadosing on Micronutrients

Thousands of people, attempting to become healthier, may be poisoning their bodies with large doses of vitamin and mineral supplements that can be dangerous.

I've never seen anything on the subject. How is one supposed to know?

That's the problem. For years we have been given minimum requirements and Recommended Daily Allowances (RDA) for most vitamins and a few of the minerals, but no safe upper limits of dosages have been established. This is because, so far, vitamins and minerals are classified under *foods* rather than *drugs,* and thus are not subjected to the extensive scrutiny and testing that drugs receive.

What kinds of damage can result from excessive intake of vitamins and minerals?

One danger is the notion that excessive doses can prevent serious diseases such as cancer, heart disease, and osteoporosis. Large supplemental doses of single nutrients may interfere with the absorption of other nutrients. For example, high levels of iron

129

appear to reduce zinc absorption, while high intakes of zinc seem to impair copper absorption.

Several vitamins are soluble only in fat. Overloads cannot be excreted, but are picked up and stored in body fat. Toxic doses of vitamin A (20 times the RDA dose) can produce throbbing headaches, dry skin with cracked lips, joint pain, and loss of hair. Pregnant women who take megadoses of vitamin A may endanger their babies.

Other fat-soluble vitamins are vitamin D, E, and K. In excessive doses (three to five times the normal dose), vitamin D may become harmful to the linings of arteries, possibly encouraging plaque formation.

The water soluble vitamins (B-complex and C) were long thought to do no harm because the body could eliminate the excesses through the urine. But that rule went out the door in 1983 when megadoses of vitamin B-6 were shown to produce disturbances in the nervous system. Excessive doses of the water soluble vitamins have been shown to cause the body to become very wasteful of these nutrients. Megadoses of vitamin C have caused kidney stones in some people.

Another worry is that the long-term effects of megadoses are unknown. We are taking chances. Indiscriminate use can amount to over-the-counter drug abuse.

What's the safest way to get vitamins and minerals?

Ideally, we should get our micronutrients from our food. Natural foods are heavily laden with vitamins and minerals in amounts and forms that allow the body to pick and choose what it needs. Once we separate nutrients from food, once we concentrate anything in the food chain, we run the risk of upsetting this natural balance.

What about people on limited food intakes, and others who pay little attention to their nutrition?

Scientists are not too concerned about people taking a daily multivitamin tablet that supplies the recommended daily allowances for several vitamins and minerals. Supplements at reasonable levels may provide assurances in marginal situations.

But don't extra vitamins help with stress and increase energy levels?

There is no documented evidence that vitamin and mineral supplements make people more energetic or have any effect on stress. These micronutrients do not function in a magical manner. In excess, they will not push the pace of the body's biological reactions any more than extra gas in the tank will make a car go faster than its engine capacity allows. Energy comes from fuel foods (carbohydrates like grains, legumes, potatoes), not from vitamins and minerals.

While we need these micronutrients to live healthily we need them in very minuscule amounts. People don't realize that they can put all the vitamins they need for a month into a thimble, easily.

EMOTIONAL HEALTH

- *Stress*
- *Depression*
- *Emotions*
- *Mind Power*

Chapter 34
Beating Burnout

Stress has come to be linked with almost every medical problem we have these days—heart attacks, hypertension, heart disease, ulcers, colitis, headaches, backaches, asthma, nervous breakdowns, even cancer. Yet, too little stress can invite disease as well, causing fatigue, boredom, restlessness, dissatisfaction, and depression. The challenge is to find a middle road between the two extremes.

What is "stress"?

Stress occurs in any situation that requires making a change. The stress involved in adjusting to some situations can produce feelings of extreme pleasure: skiing down a smooth slope, winning a race, receiving a job promotion. Other stresses may not be quite so exciting yet cause strong feelings of satisfaction: a romantic evening, praise from a coworker, a child's good report card. Still other stresses may make us weary although they are good in themselves: a wedding, or a family reunion. Then there are stresses that exhaust and depress: a job loss, legal problems, rebellious children, divorce, the death of a loved one.

Health has been called the ability to adapt to life's stresses. If so, healthy people must find ways to pace themselves by keeping their stress in positive balance.

Are stress problems getting worse?

The pace of modern life has thrown us into a kind of time warp. We are constantly urged to go now, see now, buy now, enjoy now. After all, as the ads tell us, we have only one chance in life and we'd better grab all we can.

But after a few years of grabbing, getting, going, seeing, buying, we begin to feel battered and disappointed. The inevitable *pay later* comes along: burnout, debts, poor health, depression, and loss of interest in life. It's a vicious cycle that has trapped many well-meaning men and women.

How can we protect ourselves from such a scenario?

It's difficult to seriously damage a healthy body with stress. You can help protect your body against the harmful effects of stress with a few simple *stress inoculations*. Some of the more important ones are:

- *Regular active exercise* for at least 30 minutes a day. Exercise produces endorphins, the *feel good* hormones that protect the body against stress. Sunshine and fresh air also produce endorphins, so outdoor exercise is doubly beneficial.

- *A simple, vegetarian-centered diet.* The body easily handles such a diet. The result is increased energy, efficiency, and endurance.

- *No cigarettes, alcohol, caffeine, or other harmful drugs.* These substances all chalk up substantial *pay later* debts, often beginning the next day.

- *Adequate rest.* This includes a good night's sleep and regular times for relaxation and recreation.

- *Liberal use of water inside and out.* Drink enough water to keep the urine pale (six to eight glasses a day). A hot and cold shower each morning starts your day off right.

- *Stable life anchors.* A religious faith, a loving home, a job that makes you feel worthwhile, inspiring friends, a purpose for living—these are all vaccines against stress.

- *A positive mental attitude.* Picture a very cranky man walking to work in the pouring rain, cursing all the way. What is going on inside this man? Now picture three delighted children playing in the same rain. What is going on inside these children? Who has the most stress? The difference is not in the circumstances but in the attitude toward those circumstances.

Much of life does give us a choice. Don't procrastinate! Choose to enjoy life as it goes by. Praise the sunshine and the rain. Smell the flowers, return the smiles, play with children. This approach to life costs little and avoids hangovers. It exacts no *pay later* debt. Instead, it pays generous dividends.

> *"For as he thinketh in his heart, so is he."*
> —Proverbs 23:7

Chapter 35

Dealing With Feelings

Some experts estimate that as high as 30 percent of the population of developed Western countries suffer from anxiety and depression seriously enough to need help. Billions of tranquilizers and antidepressants are gulped down each year in desperate efforts to cope. Yet the problem grows.

But aren't feelings of depression a natural part of life?

Yes, depression is a normal emotion, but it can also be a symptom of a wide variety of medical and psychological illnesses.

How do people know when they've crossed the line?

Depressions are characterized by feelings of sadness and dejection, often accompanied by lessened physical activity. Let's look at some of the more common types:

• *The Blues* often follow periods of excitement, fatigue, or other such stresses. These depressions are short and self-limiting, rarely requiring treatment.

• *Reactive* depressions result from intense life crises such as losing a loved one or a job, a divorce, moving, or a serious illness. The effect is often protective, giving time for healing to take place. Supportive measures are indicated, with more aggressive treatment if the depression is severe or prolonged.

- *Biological* depressions, on the other hand, are often inherited. They come and go, usually with no discernible cause. These depressions often respond to treatment, although they may persist for several months despite treatment.
- *Psychotic* depressions are those in which individuals lose touch with reality; they require professional care.

How can a depressed person be helped?

Diet. A simple diet of fresh, natural foods at regular intervals decreases physical stress. Eating only fresh fruit for a day or two can work wonders in clearing the mind and banishing fatigue.

Rest. Periods of quietness and calm are especially important in today's fast-paced, pressured life. As for sleep, most people do best on seven to eight hours a night.

Exercise. One of the most exciting findings of recent years has been the benefits of exercise. Regular, active physical exercise elevates mood, increases the sense of well-being, improves sleep, relieves stress, promotes health, and helps to prevent disease. A brisk one-hour walk each day will do more good for many depressed people than medication.

What else can be done for depression?

Psychological factors are important as well:

Structure. All people, whether depressed or not, need structure in their lives. Structure improves efficiency and stability.

Productivity. Humans have a basic need to do some kind of productive work, whether heading a corporation, washing a car, or cooking a meal. A depressed person, especially, needs the feeling of completion, accomplishment, and satisfaction found in doing something useful each day.

Goals. Encourage the depressed person to make a list of positive and interesting activities, and then work on one item at a time. Check each one off as it is accomplished.

Choices. Even severely depressed people can make simple, everyday choices like deciding whether to get up in the morning or stay in bed; whether to watch television all day or look for more strengthening activities; whether to dress and groom themselves or stay in a bathrobe. Such choices, made day by day, matter a great deal because they mold the future. Even people with serious mental problems can improve their ability to cope with their life situations.

Spiritual Anchors. To be worth living, life must have meaning and value, otherwise a chronic emptiness and a fluctuating sense of despair set in. Spiritual growth can bring answers to anxiety, fear, guilt, and resentment. It can restore energy and zest for living.

What about medications?

Medications may be prescribed for specific reasons, and for stated lengths of time. Chronic use can lead to dependency and/or increased depression.

Depression is no longer the fearful, discouraging, chronic affliction it once was. By improving physical health, developing positive mental attitudes, and pursuing spiritual goals, most people can deal with their feelings of depression and live rewarding and productive lives.

Emotions   Chapter 36
Endorphins: the Happy Hormones

FEEL GOOD drugs are almost irresistible. From cocaine to caffeine, people are reaching more and more for something that can help ease the numbing stress and paralyzing pressures that make up so much of modern life. But as evidence mounts that these drugs are destructive, scientists are discovering that a healthy body can make its own *feel good* substances that are both protective and health promoting.

You mean a person's body actually makes "drugs"?

Yes. If drugs are defined as chemical substances, then the body makes thousands each day. If drugs are defined as substances used as medicine to treat disease, the answer is still *yes.* The human body is engaged in constant efforts to heal itself.

What kinds of "good drugs" does the body make?

The most potent man-made "feel good" drugs are the narcotics. Narcotics block pain and produce feelings of extreme well-being. They are valuable in controlling severe, unavoidable pain, but over time they can become destructive and addictive.

More recently, scientists have found that the body produces narcotic-like substances of its own. These can be lumped together under the general term *endorphins.*

Want to see these hormones in action? The next time you stub your toe or smash your finger, notice how quickly the intense pain fades and a comforting numbness sets in. People injured in accidents and soldiers wounded in battle seldom realize at first how badly they are hurt. Athletes can even fracture bones in the heat of competition and not feel the pain until the game is over. These are examples of the body's endorphins at work.

Years ago, Dr. Hans Selye found that fear or anger could trigger a blast of adrenaline in the body. The extra adrenaline produced a surge of energy that enabled the person to either fight or flee the source of danger.

Research later demonstrated that feelings of fear and anger can harm the body if they are experienced over long periods of time. Other negative emotions such as grief, hatred, bitterness, and resentment, if prolonged, can also exhaust emergency mechanisms and weaken the body's defenses against disease.

If negative emotions can be destructive, what about positive ones?

Norman Cousins opened the door to a new field of research when he helped heal himself of a fatal, hopeless disease by using positive emotions such as joy, laughter, love, gratitude, and faith, along with sensible health practices. Since then, scientists in the field of psychoneuroimmunology have isolated many of the substances these emotions produce in the brain. They are the endorphins, and they not only block pain, but they can promote healing, strengthen the immune system, and produce wonderful feelings of well-being.

Are you saying that the way we think and feel can either damage or help heal our bodies?

Emotions are a very special part of our humanity. Clinging to persistent, negative emotions can promote disease, while nurturing positive emotions benefits every part of the body. For instance, doctors are learning that they must not shut the door of hope on terminally ill patients. The caring physician who, with confidence and optimism, tells his patient, "I have a feeling you are going to be that one person in ten who conquers this disease," will often be surprised by a fulfillment of his prophecy. This is quite different from his saying, "You have only a 10 percent chance of surviving."

How else can we encourage the production of these special hormones?

We have known for a long time that physical exercise is beneficial to health. But scientists began noticing that the good feelings which came from exercise could not be explained by their fitness effect alone. Something more was happening, and that *something more* proved to be an increase in endorphins.

Could this feeling just be a result of positive thinking?

The action of both narcotics and endorphins can be reversed by a particular chemical. A person whose pain is relieved with morphine will almost immediately lose that effect if this chemical is given. A person who is feeling a heightened sense of well-being from the body's production of endorphins will also lose that effect if the chemical is given. It's that specific.

But, yes, endorphin production is a result of positive thinking. Solving conflicts, banishing hatred and resentment, cultivating a loving, generous, thankful disposition, finding a strong faith—all these will boost the production of endorphins in our brains and strengthen the ability of the body to resist disease. And the physical benefit of a daily walk is the frosting on the cake.

Chapter 37

You Are What You Think

Aristotle once said that a healthy body and a healthy mind were somehow intertwined, but the idea has traveled a rocky road ever since.

I thought that was pretty well accepted these days!

Yes, and no.

Some scientists still question a direct link between emotion and disease, because they are not able to prove conclusively that a person's state of mind is able to cause or cure a specific disease.

What is emerging, however, is a better understanding of the body's immune system. While scientists can't take one particular emotion, such as anger, and relate it to a specific disease like a heart attack, they can now measure the body's immune response to specific stresses.

What is the immune system?

The human body is protected by millions of *fighting units,* circulating in the blood stream. These consist of different types of *soldiers,* each group having its own specific function. *Central Control* can order out new *units* when disease invades the body. During times of peace the numbers are reduced and the *fighters* become patrols. This is a simplified explanation of the immune system.

What affects the immune system?

A healthful diet, physical fitness, and positive emotional states can stimulate and strengthen the body's immune system. On the other hand, illness, drugs, and excessive stress can weaken it. AIDS occurs when the entire immune system has been decimated.

Emotions can affect it?

Very likely. Scientists report that people in depressed and negative emotional states may be especially vulnerable to diseases affecting the immune system, such as asthma, rheumatoid arthritis, and cancer.

How can feelings affect health?

Scientists call it the *placebo effect*. Perhaps the best way to explain it would be to illustrate it with a story:

Working late one night, I was nearly overcome by sleepiness.

Remembering that my secretary keeps a jar of instant coffee in her desk, I added several tablespoons of the powder to a cup of water, gulped it down, and waited.

Within 10 minutes I felt energized—yes, caffeine mobilizes blood sugar. Then came heightened alertness—yes, it also stimulates the nervous system. I rushed to the bathroom, confirming that caffeine is also a diuretic. The boost lasted the three hours I needed to finish the project.

Next morning I confessed to my secretary. She listened and began to smile.

"I'm glad my coffee helped," she said. "But didn't you notice it was *decaffeinated?*"

It worked because you thought it would work.

Yes. This *placebo effect* is commonly used to test new medicines. One group of test subjects is given the real thing, while another group receives a look-alike. Surprisingly, placebo subjects often report as good, and sometimes even better results than those who receive the actual medication.

In short, thoughts and emotions directly influence the mind which, in turn, powerfully affects the body. Reports are on record of people who believed they were going to die, and they did, though no direct cause could be found.

Will positive emotions, then, strengthen *the immune system?*

Newer studies are suggesting that a stable emotional life is as important to good health as more traditional influences such as improved diet, regular exercise, and the avoidance of alcohol, tobacco, and other drugs.

Positive emotions and sensible health practices, it appears, can stimulate the production of endorphins. These mysterious substances are manufactured by the brain and can produce remarkable feelings of well-being. Apparently they *pep up* the immune system as well. Endorphins, in other words, help make you feel better while they also help make you well.

So I can cure myself by thinking nice thoughts?

You should never neglect whatever *physical* cures exist for a health problem. Giving up smoking, watching your weight, getting regular exercise, taking medication—none of what I've said makes these things unimportant.

But in addition, keep an eye on your attitude. As King Solomon said,

"A cheerful heart is good medicine, but a crushed spirit dries up the bones."
—Proverbs 17:22 (NIV)

And Paul adds,

So, "Whatever is true, whatever is noble, whatever is right, whatever is pure, whatever is lovely, whatever is admirable—if anything is excellent or praiseworthy— think about such things."
—Philippians 4:8 (NIV)

Natural Remedies

- *Plant Food*
- *Digestion*
- *Fiber*
- *Breakfast*
- *Exercise*
- *Super Fluid*
- *Bottled? or Tap?*
- *Sunlight*
- *Tobacco*
- *Alcohol*
- *Caffeine*
- *Drugs*
- *Air*
- *Rest*
- *Trust in Divine Power*

Plant Food   Chapter 38

The Ultimate Diet

Vegetarians are sprouting up all over—more than 14 million in the United States alone. Once stereotyped as food fanatics or left-over hippies, vegetarians are now widely respected. They are considered healthier and their diet more ecologically sound.

Why go to the trouble of being a vegetarian?

Seven out of 10 Americans suffer and die prematurely of three killer diseases: heart disease, cancer, and stroke. In his comprehensive report to the nation titled *Nutrition and Health,* C. Everett Koop, MD, stated unequivocally that the Western diet was the major contributor to these diseases. He confirmed that saturated fat and cholesterol, eaten in disproportionate amounts, were the main culprits. He reminded people that animal products are the largest source of saturated fat as well as the only source of cholesterol. To compound the problem, Dr. Koop pointed out, these foods are usually eaten at the expense of complex-carbohydrate-rich foods such as grains, fruits, and vegetables.

The average risk of heart disease for a man eating meat, eggs, and dairy products is 50 percent. The risk for a man who leaves off meat is 15 percent. However, the coronary risk of a vegetarian who leaves off meat, eggs, and dairy products drops to only 4 percent.

An editorial in the *Journal of the American Medical Association* commented on these advantages, stating that a total vegetarian diet can prevent up to 90 percent of our strokes and 97 percent of our heart attacks.

Going beyond prevention, Dr. Dean Ornish published studies proving, beyond a shadow of a doubt, that a very low fat vegetarian diet could reverse heart disease in patients scheduled for coronary bypass surgery.

The risk for cancer of the prostate, breast, and colon is three to four times higher for people who consume meat, eggs, and dairy products on a daily basis when compared to those who eat them sparingly or not at all. In addition, vegetarian women have stronger bones and fewer fractures, and they lose less bone as they age.

Studies of long-lived vegetarian people like the Hunzas, who are healthy and active into advanced age, contrast sharply with the short lifespans and increased disease rates of Alaskan Eskimos, who depend largely on what they catch from the sea.

Are vegetarians able to meet their nutrient needs?

Easily. The RDA for protein is 44 to 61 grams for adults, which works out to around 10 percent of calories eaten. A beefsteak offers about 25 percent of its calories as usable protein. The protein content of most fresh vegetables averages around 20 percent of total calories, and grains usually exceed 10 percent. In addition, dried beans and peas carry close to 25 percent of calories as usable protein. So there is plenty of protein in plant foods, which are also low in fat, high in fiber and contain no cholesterol.

Studies show that complementary proteins and iron supplies are essentially nonproblems in humans eating a variety of plant foods, although *pure* vegetarians may require small supplements of vitamin B_{12}.

Will switching to a vegetarian diet affect my weight?

If you replace the meat in your diet with donuts, Twinkies, french fries and other high-fat, high-sugar morsels, then, yes, you will probably gain weight.

However, if you choose to eat more foods-as-grown, simply prepared without those nutrition-depleted calories, you can shed excess weight and stabilize at a healthier level.

What would be the ecological effects?

Shifting toward a vegetarian lifestyle would greatly ease the environmental impact of our present meat-centered diet. Pollution from animal-based agriculture is greater than from all other human and industrial activities combined. Overgrazing and intense cultivation of land for production of animal foods contributes substantially to the massive erosion and the irretrievable loss of six billion tons of valuable topsoil annually in America.

But the impact of a meat-centered diet goes beyond North America. In Central America, for example, irreparable damage with global implications continues on a daily basis. Americans eat over 200 million pounds of Central American beef every year. Powerful landowners have destroyed nearly half the region's rain forests, turning them into grazing lands for the cattle needed to supply the ever-expanding hamburger chains. Fifty-five square feet of land is needed to produce one quarter-pound hamburger.

Doesn't this effect the world's food supplies?

By moving toward vegetarianism we could use our grains and beans to feed the world's hungry people instead of the world's cattle and poultry. The amount of land needed to feed one person consuming a meat-based diet would feed 20 vegetarians. One acre of land yields 165 pounds of beef but 20,000 pounds of potatoes. To produce one pound of edible flesh from a feedlot steer requires 10 pounds of grain and soybeans. It's a poor conversion system that operates at a 10 percent efficiency level!

The evidence against meat continues to grow as it once did for cigarettes. The vegetarian diet is proving to be the ultimate diet—maximizing health, preventing disease, releasing food to the hungry, and preserving the planet. It's time for Americans to stop slaughtering nine million creatures every day for food.

OK, I'm convinced. How do I make the transition?

Some people can switch to a vegetarian diet *cold turkey,* but others do it more gradually, eliminating red meat first . . . then poultry . . . fish . . . and finally dairy products.

Another idea is to begin with one or more meatless days a week. As you experiment with vegetarian dishes, you can gradually increase the number of meatless meals.

Switching to a less meat-dependent diet is really not such a big deal. We already eat bean burritos, pasta, and other standard meatless fare. Stretch your imagination, enjoy the varied tastes, save on your food dollar, and savor a new level of health.

Digestion   Chapter 39
What Follows the Swallows

Proteins, fats, and carbohydrates are the major constituents of food. They carry the food's energy to the body. The body digests each in an orderly fashion, yet at different rates. It digests simple carbohydrates (sugars) quickly while fats take longer. Proteins and complex carbohydrates (starches) fall somewhere in between.

Is there some benefit in eating a starch food, for instance, at one meal, and a protein food at a different time?

Nature doesn't support this idea. All plant foods and some animal foods are combinations of carbohydrate, protein, and fat. Broccoli and peas, for example, contain a fair percentage of protein, and even lettuce has a little fat.

To get a pure carbohydrate meal you would need to eat white sugar or the starchy residue that's left after removing the gluten from white flour. A pure protein meal could be egg whites or dry cottage cheese curds. For the fat meal a few tablespoons of butter or cooking oil would do. *Pure foods,* in this sense, don't occur in nature, but they can be manufactured.

How does the stomach handle these different food constituents?

Digestion is the process by which the body breaks food down into its component parts so that the sugars and starches of the carbohydrates become glucose; fats become fatty acids, and proteins become amino acids. The blood can pick up these substances from the intestines.

Only a part of digestion occurs in the stomach. The rest occurs in the mouth and intestines. In an amazingly orderly fashion, carbohydrate digestion begins in the mouth with the saliva and continues in the stomach. Protein digestion begins in the stomach and continues in the intestines. Fat is digested entirely in the intestines.

Does the acidity or alkalinity of foods affect this process?

The stomach has three basic functions:

- It breaks food particles down to a more uniform size by muscular action.
- It brings the food mass to the needed consistency by adding or absorbing fluid.
- It brings the stomach contents to the necessary degree of acidity by secreting acidic digestive juices. This phase accomplishes those parts of digestion that require an acid medium.

When the stomach contents go on to the intestines, they become alkalinized by juices that the pancreas secretes. The digestive process is completed in the intestines.

Don't some foods bog down this process?

Foods high in fats are the worst offenders. The body cannot digest fats until they are alkalinized and emulsified by the intestinal juices (much as the grease on your hands cannot be removed until it is emulsified with soap and hot water). But the body has protective mechanisms which meter the fat from the stomach to the intestines so that the emulsification process isn't overwhelmed. If the amount of fat in a meal is not large, it will make little difference in digestion time. But a meal high in fat takes considerably longer to pass through the stomach.

Is there an ideal balance of foods?

The body can handle three or four kinds of whole plant foods with maximum efficiency and minimum stress. A more complex meal takes longer to digest and exacts a higher energy price from the body.

Eating snacks between meals disrupts the orderly digestive processes and stresses the stomach. Digestive problems will be slight if the stomach is presented with a simple meal, allowed to digest it, and then is given time to rest awhile before adding more food. Ideally, meals should be four or five hours apart.

You mean we shouldn't eat anything between meals?

Take a drink of water. Water requires no digestion. It passes right through, giving everything a good rinse. If you just must have something more, choose a piece of fresh fruit or munch on some raw veggies.

Fighting Fads   Chapter 40
The Rise and Fall of
Oat Bran

O nce billed as a quick fix for pulling down stubborn cholesterol levels, oat bran cut a blazing swath across public
awareness. Foodmakers jumped to take advantage of the
windfall, deciding that nearly everything went better with oat bran.
An oatmeal war broke out. Oat bran became scarce and the price
shot up.

Was there scientific evidence for the claims?

Allowing for the usual exaggerations, oat bran did appear to be
remarkably effective. In one study, for instance, a group of men with
high blood cholesterol levels were given a bowl of oat bran
cereal and five oat bran muffins each day along with their usual food.
Another group, with similar cholesterol levels, ate their usual diet.
After 10 days the oat bran group had dropped their cholesterol levels by 13 percent.

What was the secret?

The secret appeared to be in oat bran fiber. There are many kinds
of fiber, but they all fall into two basic groups: those that dissolve
in water (soluble fiber), and those that don't (insoluble fiber).

Insoluble fiber absorbs water in the intestinal tract, increases stool bulk, and helps speed the movement of food through the intestines. It has a valuable laxative effect and helps to stabilize blood sugar.

Soluble fiber, on the other hand, is the type that affects cholesterol. Cholesterol is a by-product of digestion. Without soluble fiber to help carry it out of the intestines, most of this cholesterol would be reabsorbed into the bloodstream, adding to the already high levels found in most Westerners. It was believed that oat bran fiber had an exceptionally high affinity for these cholesterol by-products.

Sounds good. Was there a problem with that?

The prestigious *New England Journal of Medicine* published a study several months later that appeared to pull the rug out from under the hype. The mighty oat, it suddenly seemed, was not what it was cracked up to be. Besides, people were getting tired of oat bran mush. Even the muffins were becoming a bore.

So it was just another fad!

Not altogether. The new study didn't debunk oat bran as a food. Instead, it demonstrated that oat bran didn't act in the way people presumed it did. It was not a *magical potion* which could be gulped down to ream out the blood vessels or sprinkled on harmful foods to make them okay.

What the study showed was that a big bowl of any hot starchy cereal, eaten for breakfast, would displace an appreciable amount of bacon, eggs, sausage, *croissants,* and other foods that kick in the liver's cholesterol-producing machinery.

And other studies demonstrated that, while eating soluble fiber might lower cholesterol levels, oat-bran fiber held no advantage over the soluble fibers in other foods, such as beans and fruit.

These observations make sense. Any dietary change where low-fat, starchy, no-cholesterol plant foods replace high-fat, high-cholesterol animal foods has been repeatedly shown to be effective in lowering cholesterol levels.

You're confusing me!

People who eat lots of plant foods will get all the fiber they need, both soluble and insoluble. However, for people unable or unwilling to follow such a diet, adding oat and other brans to their food is a helpful step.

The moral of all this? It's folly to focus excessively on a single food or nutrient. While sensationalized *discoveries* and simplistic *solutions* to complex health problems are the darlings of the media and the advertisers, the oat debacle should enlarge our understanding of the role that the wide variety of available plant foods play in promoting health. Grains in almost any form make for healthful eating. But to eat largely of a single extract, such as oat bran, produces a lopsided diet.

Studies over the years have demonstrated that a high-fiber, low-fat, meatless diet will lower cholesterol levels from 20 percent to 35 percent in four to eight weeks for most people. Adding oat bran to such a diet contributes little.

Oats and oat bran are nutritious, health-promoting foods. They should be part of a well-balanced diet. But preoccupation with exciting new discoveries and the eternal desire for the *quick fix* continue to encourage extreme and impractical solutions to real health problems.

A balanced, healthful lifestyle may not grab headlines or create profitable new markets, but it brings improved health that lasts.

               Chapter 41

Jumpstart Your Day

Many people can't face food when they crawl out of bed. A quick cup of coffee is a standard adult breakfast. An increasing number of children arrive at school having eaten nothing at all.

Why bother with breakfast?

A group of scientists spent ten years studying the effects of different kinds of breakfasts versus no breakfast at all on people of different ages.

A good breakfast, they concluded, can help both children and adults be less irritable, more efficient, and more energetic.

More recent studies have even linked healthy breakfasts with less chronic disease, increased longevity, and better health.

A *good breakfast,* by the way, is one that provides at least one-third of the day's calories. Start your day with a whole-grain cereal, whole-grain bread, and a couple of whole, fresh fruits, and you'll find that your energy level stays high throughout the morning.

What's wrong with orange juice and a Danish?

You need something with more fiber in it. Although fiber isn't digested by the body, it does absorb water as it moves through the stomach and intestines. The resulting spongy mass acts as a gentle barrier to the food particles suspended in it so that they are not absorbed too quickly.

On the other hand, fiberless foods, especially sugared foods and drinks, quickly pass into the bloodstream, and cause blood sugar levels to rapidly rise and fall. That helps explain why your energy and efficiency drop off in the later morning hours when little or no fiber-containing foods are eaten at breakfast.

But I'm not hungry until mid-morning!

Probably the biggest reason people feel that way is that they eat a large meal in the evening. (TV snacks don't help either!) When they go to bed, their stomachs are still busy digesting all that food. But the stomach needs rest, too. An exhausted stomach does not feel like taking on a big breakfast.

The solution?

- Eat a light supper at least four hours before bedtime, or even skip supper a few times.
- Eat or drink nothing but water or fruit between supper and bed-time.

If you do these two things, you'll be ready to break the fast of the long night.

Won't skipping breakfast help me lose weight?

Surprisingly, no. The Iowa Breakfast Studies demonstrated that the omission of breakfast does not have an advantage in weight reduction. It's actually a disadvantage because those who omit break-fast accentuate their hunger and eat more snacks and food the rest of the day to make up for the lack. They also suffer a significant loss of efficiency in the late morning hours.

But I don't have time to eat breakfast.

Many people are in the habit of staying up late, then sleeping in as long as they can in the morning. Although a few people work more efficiently at night, most don't fit that timetable.

Try going to bed early enough so you can wake up in the morning feeling refreshed and with time to spare. Begin the day by drinking a glass or two of water to rinse and freshen your stomach. Pull on your gym clothes and get some active exercise, like a brisk walk. Shower and dress for the day. Then fix and eat a hot breakfast.

This works with children, too. Put them to bed early enough so that they wake up in time to join the family around the breakfast table.

A good breakfast boosts your energy, increases your attention span and heightens your sense of well-being. You'll be less apt to cheat on your diet by snacking. And you'll be in better control of your emotions.

What a great way to start your day!

BREAKFAST CHOICES				
	Calories	Fat (gm)	Salt (mg)	Chol. (mg)
AMERICAN				
Bacon (3 sl.)	129	12	574	60
Scrambled Eggs (3)	330	24	1230	675
Hash Browns (1 C)	355	18	3265	0
Danish Roll (1)	274	15	595	35
Hot Cocoa (1 C)	213	9	295	25
Orange Juice (1 C)	120	0	6	0
TOTAL	**1,421**	**78**	**5,965**	**795**
OPTIMAL				
7 Grain Cereal (1C)	159	1	400	
Banana (1)	95	0	3	0
NF Milk (1 C)	88	0	318	0
Grapefruit (1/2)	66	0	5	0
Tofu (1 C)	118	7	1233	0
H. Browns, no oil (1 C)	101	0	22	0
W. W. Bread (1 sl.)	61	1	330	0
TOTAL	**688**	**9**	**2,351**	**0**

Exercise — Chapter 42
Today's Fountain of Youth

The fabled Fountain of Youth lured ancient adventurers into a lifetime of fruitless searching. In time it became a symbol for an impossible dream. That was yesterday. Today, science seems able to put at least part of this dream within reach of nearly all of us.

What do you mean?

When the explorers were searching for a secret spring that would maintain perpetual youth, many people were dying in early adulthood of infectious diseases. Today, improved sanitation and hygiene, along with antibiotics, have almost eliminated those diseases. The battle has now shifted to degenerative diseases. These are the maladies that are now robbing us of our energy, disabling us prematurely, and killing us s-l-o-w-l-y.

The good news is that greater vitality, better health, and longer life can be ours through regular, brisk physical activity.

Do you mean EXERCISE? Can it really do all that?

Take a look at the facts. The adage *Use it or lose it* applies not only to muscles and bones but also to hearts, lungs, brains, blood vessels, joints, and every other part of the body. A sedentary lifestyle is a direct route to an earlier death. Inactivity kills us—literally.

A strong genetic inheritance helps some people survive incredible odds. But just living longer isn't today's only concern. People are looking for energy, good health, usefulness, and quality of life along with their lengthened years.

Just how does physical exercise help us live longer and better?

Here are some of the ways:

- Exercise helps you FEEL GOOD! Life becomes more fun, and the *high* that comes from exercise won't let you down later. Moreover, the hormones producing the exercise high are proving to be health promoting as well.

- Exercise strengthens the heart. This is important in a culture in which every second person dies of heart and vascular disease.

- Exercise lowers blood pressure and resting heart rate, protecting the heart and blood vessels.

- Exercise lowers LDL cholesterol levels in the blood and often raises HDL cholesterol, again decreasing heart and vascular risk. (LDL is the bad part of cholesterol; HDL the good part.)

- Exercise strengthens bones by helping retain calcium and other important minerals. Sedentary people past age 40 increasingly lose calcium and bone mass.

- Exercise lifts depression. Outdoor exercise is one of the most valuable tools for fighting this common and disabling malady.

- Exercise relieves anxiety and stress. In our harried, pressured society, physical activity is proving to be an effective antidote.

- Exercise increases overall energy and efficiency in all areas of our lives.

- Exercise helps maintain desirable weight levels. It builds muscles and burns fat. Moderate exercise blunts appetite by temporarily increasing blood sugar levels.

- Exercise improves circulation, and that makes for clearer minds, better sleep, and faster healing of damaged body areas.

What kind of exercise are you talking about? Not everyone can jog, or run marathons.

Every one of these listed benefits can come from plain, simple walking. Walking is the ideal exercise. It's inexpensive. It's safe. Nearly everyone can do it. And it's fun! You can select your own speed and stop when you want. As your fitness improves you can gradually add speed and time.

Other good exercises are swimming, bicycling, gardening, yard work, and golf—if you leave the carts behind. For hardier souls, jogging, stair climbing, rock climbing, jumping rope, and snow skiing provide challenging variations. In bad weather try stationary bicycles, trampolines, rowing machines, or simply walking or jogging in place. To be effective, active (aerobic) exercise should be brisk and continuous for at least 15 to 20 minutes. Most people can work up to this goal. A daily program of 30 to 40 minutes of active exercise will give you maximum benefits. To control weight, increase the time to one hour. You can divide the hour into two or three sessions if you wish.

Is it true that reaching a certain pulse rate is necessary for exercise to be effective?

There are exercise regimes for specific purposes. The concept of *training heart rate* is particularly useful in strengthening the heart. Weight training is also proving valuable. But remember: even moderate activities, such as brisk walking, will improve fitness and lower the risk of heart attack as much as 30 percent. Every step counts.

But I hate to exercise. It's boring!

We all do many boring things every day: brushing teeth, cleaning the house, washing the car, mowing the lawn, doing dishes, going to work. But we do these things because we like the rewards: beautiful teeth, an attractive home, a clean car, a regular paycheck. After awhile these activities become routine, an accepted part of our daily living.

Let's look at exercise the same way. Its benefits are far greater than a clean house—they will last a lifetime.

Super Fluid — Chapter 43

The No-Calorie Wonder

Forcing the body to work with limited amounts of fluid is like trying to wash the dinner dishes in a cupful of water. When you don't drink enough water, the body must excrete wastes in a much more concentrated form, causing body odor, bad breath, and unpleasant-smelling urine.

Don't most people drink plenty of water?

Surprisingly, the average person today drinks more soft drinks and alcohol than water. And not far behind are coffee and milk.

Notice what happens next time you go to a restaurant for a meal. You will usually be served a large glass of ice water and then asked expectantly, "And what would you like to drink?"

Why does it matter what beverages I drink? They all contain water, don't they?

The body uses water in all forms, but beverages can pose special problems. Many have calories that must be digested like food. These calories may produce extra fat storage, swings in blood sugar, and slowed digestion. Water alone, on the other hand, goes right through the stomach whether or not food is there. It requires no processing, no digesting, does not irritate or disturb body functions, and it has no calories.

Sugar in beverages requires extra water for metabolism. Most beverages increase acid secretion in the stomach. Cola drinks contain phosphorus, a chemical that can help deplete the body's calcium supplies, contributing to brittle bones.

Do the "no sugar" diet drinks solve the problems?

Diet beverages don't contain sugar, but they present other concerns. Nearly all beverages, sugared or not, contain chemicals that are added for color, flavor, preservation, and other reasons. Some of these may irritate delicate stomach linings, and some may also require the liver and kidneys to detoxify and dispose of them.

Drinking *water* eliminates these problems. No extra calories to slow down digestion or add unwanted fat, no irritants to stress sensitive linings of the digestive tract, and fewer foreign chemicals to threaten delicate body machinery.

How much water should I drink?

Enough to keep the urine pale. The body loses about 10 to 12 cups of water a day through the skin, lungs, urine, and feces. Food provides two to four cups of water, leaving us six to eight glasses of water to drink.

Get into the habit of drinking water liberally. Drink on arising, in mid-morning, mid-afternoon, and early evening. A drink of water is like an internal shower—it rinses the stomach and prepares it for its work.

So start the day right. Give that early morning drink some zest by adding a twist of lemon. Then during morning and afternoon *coffee breaks,* reach for a glass of water and drink to your body's content. In the evening, drink away some of your sleepiness and the temptation to snack.

Water is exactly what the body needs to carry out all its life processes. It's the perfect beverage, and one of life's greatest blessings.

The next time you are asked, "Anything to drink?" you can say, "Yes, a glass of water is fine. In fact, it's perfect."

Bottled? or Tap?   Chapter 44
Designer Water

What with reports of contamination by heavy metals, nuclear wastes, fertilizers, pesticides, herbicides, and leaking fuels—not to mention the sorry state of some public water supply systems—some people are afraid to drink the water that comes out of their kitchen faucet.

What are some alternatives to tap water?

• *Bulk waters* sold in one-gallon plastic jugs are the most popular. These come from springs or wells, or are processed from ordinary tap water.

• *Mineral waters* contain dissolved minerals, sometimes natural, sometimes added. There are no upper limits set for the amount of minerals that can be put in.

• *Sparkling water* is a generic term for any carbonated water. Some, like club sodas, are relatively high in sodium and should not be used by people with high blood pressure.

• *Seltzer water* refers to filtered, carbonated tap water that has no added mineral salts. Many, however, have added sugars, up to 100 calories per eight ounces.

• *Distilled water* is the purest. All minerals have been removed, either by distillation or by osmosis, leaving the water tasting rather flat. It's the hardness of the water—the minerals—that give water its flavor.

Is bottled water safer or better tasting than that from the tap?

A lot of people must think so. Last year Americans spent nearly one billion dollars on bottled waters!

You should know, however, that federal and state requirements for bottled water are exactly the same as they are for tap water. If your water supply is up to standard, what comes out of your faucet may be just as pure, just as safe, and just as wholesome as the water you buy in a grocery store.

As a matter of fact, according to several research centers, most of the ordinary tap water sampled in North America proved to be as good or better than most bottled waters. In one comparative taste sampling, water samples from New York, Los Angeles, Tucson, Memphis, and Atlantic City tasted better than most *mountain spring* bottled water sold over the counter.

Are you saying that most tap water is safe to drink?

It's true that some water supplies have been chemically contaminated. It's also true that outbreaks of infectious diseases have been traced to tap water—though this is extremely rare in developed countries today. But we need to keep this in perspective. Many people fear flying, even though statistics show that they are safer in an airplane than in a bus, train, automobile, or even crossing a street. Likewise, any problem with a water supply is apt to be broadcast out of all proportion to the real danger it poses to the majority of people.

How can I tell if my tap water is safe?

There are a number of ways to protect yourself:

- Public water systems are checked for safety, sometimes several times a day. The test results are public property, and you can request a copy.

- If you suspect possible contamination between your municipal supply and your home, you should have your water tested at the point of its use.
- If you are among the 40 percent of Americans who depend on private wells, your local government may test your water for a nominal fee. National mail order testing services are also available.

What can I do if my tap water is unsafe?

If you live in an area with unsafe water, you can protect yourself by installing your own filtering system. (An under-the-counter device may be all you need.) A good charcoal filter removes most contaminants and makes the water taste good. Other more sophisticated methods are also available.

There are simpler solutions as well. The dangers of lead poisoning can be minimized by running the tap for a minute or so before drinking from it. As for chlorine, draw water into an open pitcher or a glass jar and let it stand. The chlorine will evaporate, and the taste will improve.

This all seems so complicated. No wonder some people fear their drinking water!

The irony is that most of us face more health hazards from not drinking enough water than we do from its possible contaminants. Tap water is hundreds of times cheaper than bottled, and it's nearly always at our fingertips. If it checks out safe, we should not fear drinking it. Just make sure to drink plenty of it—six to eight glasses a day.

Sunlight

Kiss of the Sun

Excessive exposure to sunlight can cause skin cancer as well as premature wrinkling and aging of the skin. In proper amounts, however, the sun's rays can be good for your health.

What are some of the good things about sunlight?

A lot!

To begin with, sunlight kills germs. That's why it is important to sun and air out blankets, quilts, and other items that are not washed regularly and sterilized in an automatic dryer.

Proper amounts of sunshine also give the skin a healthy glow and help make it smooth and pliable. A moderately tanned skin is more resistant to infections and sunburns than untanned skin.

Then too, sunlight elevates the mood for most people, producing a sense of well-being. (Just don't stay out too long and get sunburned!) Combined with active exercise, sunshine is an important adjunct in treating acute and chronic depressions. Remember, when depressed during winter's cold and gloomy months, try to catch any possible ray of sunshine.

What's more, the body is able to manufacture vitamin D by the action of sunlight on the skin. Vitamin D enables the body to pick up calcium from the intestines for use in building healthy bones. It prevents both childhood and adult rickets and aids in the prevention of osteoporosis.

Sunlight also helps:

- enhance the immune system
- alleviate pain from swollen arthritic joints
- relieve certain symptoms of PMS.

Some reports suggest that sunlight may also help lower blood cholesterol levels.

And the bad ones?

Sunlight is a major risk factor for skin cancer, especially in light-skinned people. Too much sunlight, for them, may be particularly damaging.

You should also know that burning the skin is extremely harmful for everyone. Every burn destroys healthy, living tissue. Repeated burns cause irreversible damage and can set up a person for skin cancer.

And if all that isn't bad enough, repeated sunburn and even repeated deep tanning of the skin gradually destroy its elasticity and its oil glands, producing wrinkling and premature aging.

Some recent studies suggest that a high-fat diet, when combined with exposure to sunlight, may also promote cancers of the skin.

What are some guidelines for safe, healthy exposure to sunlight?

- Modest tanning is protective, like putting sunglasses on your skin. But you must understand your own tolerance to sunlight. Fair-skinned people and redheads may have to begin with only five minutes of exposure to the sun per day. Darker-skinned people can begin with 10 to 15 minutes per day. Up to 30 minutes of sunshine, exposed to as much of the body as possible, is a realistic goal for most people.

• Never, never burn! Wear protective clothing, eyewear and a protective sunscreen if needed. Be especially careful around snow or water and on cloudy days.

• If you have an outdoor trip or vacation coming up, prepare your skin by giving it progressive exposure in the days beforehand, to the point of pinking up.

• A few minutes of sunshine on your face and hands each day will produce all the vitamin D you need.

• Open up your house to the sunshine each morning. It will improve your health and lift your spirits.

For thousands of years, sunlight has been known as a mediator of life. But we know today that it can be healing or destructive; it can be the kiss of life or the kiss of death, depending on how we use it.

Deadliest Drug
in the World

Smoking is not only hazardous to your health—it can be hazardous to your job prospects as well. Twice as many smokers are out of work as nonsmokers. Though few will admit it, most employers would reject a smoker competing for a job with an equally qualified nonsmoker.

Don't you think the risks of smoking are being exaggerated?

No way! For example, smokers at Dow Chemical, when compared to nonsmokers, had six days more absenteeism, eight days more disability and 12 percent more illness, costing the company $1,900 to $2,300 more per smoker per year.

The hard facts consistently point to tobacco as the deadliest drug in the world. Last year it killed 430,000 Americans—more than all who died from AIDS, street drugs, fires, car crashes, and homicides combined. It also kills thousands more *involuntary smokers*—persons forced to breathe *second-hand* smoke.

How does smoking cause lung cancer?

Normally your lungs' air passages are lined with millions of tiny hairs called cilia. The cilia act like little brooms, protecting the air

173

tubes by sweeping dusts, tar, and other foreign materials gradually upward, like escalators, until they can be spit out.

Every time a blast of tobacco smoke hits these cilia, however, they slow down, and soon stop moving. As a result, the trapped tars from the tobacco smoke begin boring into the cells lining the air tubes. Over time, this constant irritation turns some of the cells cancerous.

This transformation takes many years. But once it begins, the cancer steadily eats its way deeper into the lung. By the time it is discovered, it's usually too late.

Is lung cancer the leading cause of death in smokers?

No. Tobacco causes 115,000 lung cancer deaths per year in the United States. In contrast, smoking is responsible for 30 percent of coronary heart deaths, some 165,000, plus at least 33,000 fatal strokes.

The nicotine and carbon monoxide in tobacco smoke are the main culprits that promote vascular disease. While nicotine produces the sensation of soothing relaxation and well-being—smoking's main appeal it also constricts small arteries, depriving the heart, brain, lungs and other important areas of vital oxygen. Nicotine is also addictive.

Carbon monoxide interferes directly with the ability of red blood cells to carry oxygen. This causes shortness of breath, lack of endurance, and promotes and accelerates narrowing and hardening of the arteries.

That's a lot of bad news. Is there more?

Unfortunately there is a lot more.

- Smokers have much more cancer of the mouth, larynx, esophagus, pancreas, bladder, kidneys, and cervix than do nonsmokers.
- Emphysema gradually destroys lung tissue, producing death by suffocation. In the United States 60,000 of these grisly deaths occur each year as a result of smoking.
- Ulcers of the stomach and duodenum are 60 percent more common in smokers.

- Smoking pulls calcium out of the skeleton, accelerating the bone-thinning process known as osteoporosis.
- Smoking during pregnancy has an adverse effect on fetal development and increases the risk of death after birth up to 35 percent.

If a person has smoked heavily for a long time, does it pay to quit?

More than 80 percent of lung cancers and 50 percent of bladder cancers could be prevented if people simply stopped smoking.

Smokers who quit begin to heal almost immediately. As the nicotine and carbon monoxide leave the body, the smoking-related risk for heart disease decreases dramatically. Although the risk for cancer decreases more slowly, the danger lessens as the weeks and months go by.

There are other payoffs to quitting: a sense of victory, increased self-esteem, pleasant breath, better tasting food, increased endurance, improved health and energy, a feeling of well-being and freedom from an inconvenient, unpopular, costly habit. Quitting may also open the way to more job opportunities.

Americans often overreact to the most trivial of risks while ignoring much more substantial threats to their health and safety. For example, more than 30 percent of regular smokers will die from some disease connected with their habit. They will also lose an average of 8.3 years from their normal life expectancy, or 12 minutes for every cigarette smoked. But many people react more forcefully to evidence of a one-in-a-million risk of getting cancer from chemicals found in drinking water!

It's time to get life back into perspective. The biggest favor you can do for your body is to kick the habit and freely breathe clean air again.

"Do you not know that your body is a temple? . . . therefore honor God with your body." —1 Cor. 6:19, 20 (NIV)

Chapter 47
The Cooler Delusion

They look like soft drinks, taste like soft drinks, and are sold like soft drinks. But there the similarity stops. These drinks contain more alcohol than a beer or a glass of wine, and they carry more calories.

Are you talking about wine coolers? They look so attractive, so healthy!

That's the strategy. Coolers come in a rainbow of colors that people associate with fruit juices. In fact, the containers and carrying packs are often plastered with pictures of fresh fruit, even though some contain no fruit or fruit juice at all.

What's more, coolers taste sweet and fizzy, like soft drinks. The alcohol taste is disguised, making them attractive to people who do not ordinarily drink alcohol. Then, too, coolers are not packaged like other types of alcoholic beverages, but like soft drinks.

Do coolers carry less risk than other alcoholic beverages?

The worst part of the cooler caper is the illusion that coolers are low in alcohol. They're not. Coolers average six percent alcohol by volume, whereas beers average four percent.

And because coolers typically come in 12-oz. bottles, the amount of alcohol in a serving can exceed that of a gin and tonic (with one ounce of liquor) or a glass of wine served at dinner.

How are coolers affecting today's young people?

Teens, especially teenage girls, are attracted to coolers. They like the name, which suggests a light, refreshing drink. And they like the taste. "Coolers are a hazard for kids because they're so easy to drink," says Diane Purcell of Chicago's Parkside Medical Services. "You can go from lemonade to a lemon cooler in one easy step. You don't have to acquire a taste for alcohol."

How serious is alcohol use among teens?

A recent survey revealed that at least 40 percent of sixth graders, and up to 80 percent of junior and senior high school students have tried wine coolers. Thirty-seven percent of all 12 through 17-year-olds currently use alcohol. And 5 million American teens already have serious problems stemming from alcohol use.

Are these kids in danger of becoming adult alcoholics?

Many kids are already alcoholics by the time they reach adulthood. Others are well on their way.

When it comes to alcohol, people carry their habits into adult life. And there are already 10.5 million adult alcoholics and 7.6 million more who have drinking-related problems. Half of all fatal auto accidents involve alcohol, as do a growing number of air fatalities. Unless we can help our teenagers, things aren't going to get better.

Alcohol exacts a heavy price from personal health. Alcohol promotes high blood pressure and is directly toxic to heart muscle. Alcohol increases the risk of stroke, sudden death from heart arrhythmias and diseased heart muscle, congestive heart failure, cirrhosis, and cancer. Alcohol also increases morbidity and hospitalization and reduces the drinker's years of useful life. And it ravages the lives of family and friends.

Perhaps the saddest statistics to emerge in recent years are those of damaged babies who are permanently retarded due to their parents' alcohol use.

What can be done to protect our young people?

Wine coolers are big business. They account for 25 percent of the industry's sales—a cool $1.7 billion.

Their attractiveness could be limited, however, if coolers—

- Were clearly labeled as alcoholic beverages, not for sale to anyone under 21.
- Had large warning labels attached that warned of the health hazards associated with drinking alcoholic beverages.
- Were subject to extra taxes, thus adding another small barrier to their availability.

And most important of all, young people who grow up in non-alcoholic homes are statistically less inclined to have problems when they reach adulthood. There is no influence more powerful than that of a good parental example.

> *"Wine is a mocker and beer a brawler; whoever is led astray by them is not wise."*
> —Proverbs 20:1 (NIV)

Caffeine

Chapter 48
Wired!

Nine out of ten North Americans take a psychotropic (mind-stimulating) drug daily. The culprit?—Everyday, ordinary, over-the-counter caffeine.

How can that be? Explain.

Do you know many people who don't drink at least one cup of coffee a day? Or tea? Or take an *extra strength* pain reliever? Or guzzle down a cola? Although caffeine-free sodas are available, they are favored mainly for children and for people with medical problems that are affected by caffeine.

But I need a lift now and then! And caffeine *isn't addictive, is it?*

An addictive substance produces observable and measurable physical and mental effects when it is withdrawn. In this sense, even small doses of caffeine, taken regularly over time, will usually produce some degree of addiction.

A good way to check yourself is to stop all caffeine intake for a few days. The most common physical withdrawal symptom is headache, varying from mild to severe. Sometimes a migraine is triggered. Other physical manifestations include feelings of exhaustion, lack of appetite, nausea, and vomiting. Symptoms last one to five days.

Psychological withdrawal can be even harder. Depression may occur. People become accustomed to reaching for the *pick-me-up* throughout the day. The urge can be compared to the desire for a cigarette—it may be difficult to resist.

Does caffeine damage the body?

• Most obvious is an over-stimulated nervous system with tremors, nervousness, anxiety, and problems with sleep. In time these symptoms give way to chronic fatigue, lack of energy, and persistent insomnia.

• Caffeinated beverages can cause stomach irritation. While additives are primarily responsible for this effect, caffeine itself has a constricting effect on blood vessels. It can thus interfere with digestion. High doses of caffeine induce vomiting.

• Caffeinated drinks also stimulate the stomach to excrete excessive acid, producing a rebound effect. This aggravates ulcers and other stomach problems.

• Caffeine has been found to interfere with calcium and iron absorption. With increasing concern over osteoporosis and anemia, these are factors to consider.

• Caffeine raises blood sugar levels, which, along with its mind-stimulating action, produces increased energy. While this seems desirable, the increased blood sugar level draws out an insulin response which not only cancels the surge, but produces a letdown. This letdown triggers the yo-yo syndrome—reaching for another caffeinated drink, and then another, and yet another.

There is more.

• Caffeine irritates the kidneys, causing diuresis (increased urine output). Some studies have linked cancers of the urinary tract to caffeine use. Caffeine has been also shown to precipitate asthmatic attacks and stir up allergies.

Are there some healthful alternatives to the caffeine high?

When you get up in the morning, follow your hot shower with a blast of cold water and towel off briskly.

At work, stand up, stretch, and take a few deep breaths every hour or so. Take a brisk walk at break time or during lunch hour. Drink a cup of cold (or hot) water several times a day. Rub a coworker's back and ask for a return favor. Walk to a window and relax your eyes on the distant landscape. Tidy up your work area. All these good things will make you feel better. Look for other creative ways to get a lift without the letdown.

In a crisis, would just a little caffeine really matter?

Occasional small doses of caffeine will hardly make a difference. The trouble is, most of us have a hard time knowing when to stop.

Chapter 49

Spiders and Sledgehammers

The way some people use drugs makes no more sense than using a sledgehammer to kill a spider. Most people don't realize that common, over-the-counter drugs can have unpleasant—even dangerous—side effects.

You must be exaggerating.

I wish I were! Take something as common as aspirin, for instance. Many people down it at the least sign of a headache, flu, or fever. Every 24 hours, as a matter of fact, Americans consume 45 tons of this drug!

Yet every year, 10,000 people will be severely poisoned by aspirin or a related product. What's more, aspirin is known to promote stomach ulcers and has been associated with Reye's syndrome, an often fatal disease in children.

Acetaminophen, another common painkiller, can cause skin rashes and even—in extreme cases—kidney and liver damage.

But prescription drugs are safe when you follow directions, right?

In the medical world, new and more effective wonder drugs are being discovered and introduced almost daily, while older ones are improved and refined. Yet the *perfect drug* still eludes us—the one that will do its job with absolutely no deleterious side effects.

Consider blood pressure drugs, for example. They are the most widely used prescription medications on the market and among the most effective. Yet they carry a host of side effects, which can include weakness, fatigue, drowsiness, headache, mental depression, dizziness, bloating, sweating, indigestion, unstable emotional states, slurred speech, raised cholesterol levels, and impotence. People who need these drugs often must test several different kinds before they find one they can tolerate.

The point is, no drug is *completely* safe. Even life-saving antibiotics carry potential problems such as: nausea, vomiting, diarrhea, and allergic reactions.

Why then are people so anxious to take drugs?

While most of today's diseases respond to lifestyle measures (such as a better diet and regular exercise), doctors who advocate these principles often find themselves rowing upstream. People are impatient; they want quick fixes rather than real solutions. If one doctor doesn't produce the desired prescription, they often seek another who will.

Simply put, people today too often want to believe there is a magic potion for their particular problem. We've an almost childlike faith that drugs can help us pep up, calm down, regulate weight, and ward off almost every conceivable ailment.

So why risk taking any drug?

Anyone taking a drug must always balance *risk* against *need.* If you have a serious bacterial infection, for instance, the risk you run by taking an antibiotic is outweighed by the risk you run if you don't take it.

If you have a tension headache, on the other hand, you'd probably be better off taking a brisk walk or a nap.

What are some guidelines for using drugs intelligently?

A good rule of thumb is to reserve drugs for specific, identifiable needs that can't be met by lesser measures. Don't use a *big-gun* medicine like antibiotics, for instance, for a *fly-swatter* problem like a head cold.

Likewise, a warm bath or a cup of herbal tea is better than a sleeping pill if you can't get to sleep. And if you don't *want* to go to sleep, a cold shower or a brisk walk is better for you than a *wake-up* pill.

When you *do* take a drug, be sure you know exactly what it's supposed to do. Understand its risks and side effects, how and when to take it, and the signs of overdosage. Don't mix medicines, and don't risk psychological dependence or physical addiction by taking any drug longer than needed. If you have more than one doctor, make sure your main doctor knows all the medications you are taking.

In short, give drugs the respect they deserve. Save them for times when they are truly needed. It's time to stop hitting spiders with sledgehammers.

Air   Chapter 50

When Breathing May Be Hazardous

Houseplants do a lot more than enhance the appearance of our homes and offices. They enrich the air with oxygen, absorb carbon dioxide, and some even remove toxic pollutants from the air we breathe.

You mean harmful pollutants can collect indoors?

Increasingly so. Many modern homes and office buildings are tightly sealed to save energy costs. But this advantage may be offset by poor ventilation and potential accumulation of indoor air pollutants.

Tobacco smoke, of course, is the most dangerous pollutant, but there are others.

Formaldehyde, for example, seeps from certain wood products, and other chemical fumes come from carpeting, copy machines, upholstery, cleaning products, and freshly dry-cleaned clothes. Carbon monoxide and nitrogen dioxide, two poisonous gases, may come from gas, oil and coal furnaces, gas ranges, fireplaces, and kerosene heaters.

Other problems occur from dust, air mites, molds and fungi, ozone, lead, asbestos, pesticide residues, and in some areas, radon gas.

How do these pollutants affect people?

Symptoms range from burning eyes, sore throats, coughing and itching, to headaches, sluggishness, nausea, dizziness, feelings of exhaustion, and depression. This cluster of symptoms is sometimes referred to as "sick building syndrome."

What can people do to protect themselves?

There are two basic ways to protect ourselves, not 100 percent, but significantly.

First, we can *control exposure.* For example:

- Ban smoking indoors. Even second-hand smoke contains hundreds of harmful chemicals.
- Make sure all gas, oil, and kerosene- and coal-burning heaters and appliances are properly vented to the outdoors, as well as coal- and wood-burning furnaces and fireplaces. And don't forget gas cooking ranges and clothes dryers.
- Keep heating and air-conditioning units well maintained. Clean air ducts and filters regularly.
- Keep chimneys open and in good repair.
- Use air fresheners, moth crystals, etc., sparingly.
- Avoid idling a vehicle in an attached garage or near an open window.

Second, we can *improve ventilation.*

The most obvious solution to indoor pollution problems is to open windows and set up good cross ventilation. Fresh air not only dilutes trapped fumes, thus decreasing their health threats, but enriches stale air as well. People often don't realize that in closed areas the same air can be breathed and rebreathed, over and over. The oxygen content decreases, and the carbon dioxide and other wastes increase, resulting in sleepiness, sluggishness, and headaches.

Here are some suggestions:

- Set air conditioners and heating systems to bring in 20-35 percent (or more) fresh air. Energy costs will be somewhat higher but health benefits will more than compensate for this.
- Air out your house at least once a day. On smoggy days, air out the house at night or in the early mornings. In most areas smog particulate matter drops considerably once the sun has set.

- Sleep with an open window. Set up cross ventilation in your bedroom if possible. You'll wake up feeling refreshed.

What about air-cleaning machines?

These machines can be expensive, complicated, messy, and most have a limited range. However, people with allergies and certain lung ailments often find them helpful. And we recommend them for anyone exposed to air polluted with tobacco smoke at home or at work.

How does air relate to personal health?

Air is composed of about 20 percent oxygen, the rest being nitrogen along with a few other gases. Since the human body operates on oxygen, each one of its 100 trillion cells must receive steady, fresh supplies, or die. Oxygen is picked up in the lungs from the air we breathe, and delivered to our bodies via the red blood cells. Well-oxygenated cells are healthy and contribute to overall well-being. Anything that diminishes oxygen supplies to the lungs, or its delivery to body cells, is detrimental.

Air molecules can also be positively or negatively charged. Polluted air is usually full of positive ions. It's commonly found on freeways, at airports, and in closed, poorly ventilated areas.

Air containing an abundance of negative ions is plentiful around lakes, in forests, near rivers and waterfalls, at the seashore, and after a rain storm. This kind of air is refreshing and gives people a lift.

Another "feel good" technique is to stop where you are and take a few slow, deep breaths several times a day. This gives your body an extra "shot of oxygen" and helps unload carbon dioxide.

Yet another way to flush your body with oxygen is to exercise. Activity opens up blood vessels and speeds those oxygen-laden red blood cells on their rounds.

And remember the houseplants. Placing at least one plant for every 100 square feet of indoor space is recommended. Live plants not only "eat" many toxic pollutants and freshen the air with oxygen, they probably slip in some extra negative ions as well!

Rest   Chapter 51
How Much Is Enough?

Life today is fast paced, exciting—and exhausting. Insomnia is epidemic. People are gulping down millions of sedatives and tranquilizers, desperate for rest that will restore their energies.

Why am I always tired?

You may have an illness, such as a cold or the flu, that is sapping your energy. Or you may be depressed.

Many otherwise healthy people, however, work in confining sedentary jobs with deadline pressures and emotionally draining problems. These people are not likely to feel rested when they get out of bed in the morning.

In addition, few people get through a day anymore without a pick-me-up, usually coffee, tea, or cola. Caffeine is a central nervous system stimulant and a common cause of insomnia.

What about chronic fatigue?

Besides tiredness and a lack of energy there is also an increase in irritability. Tempers get short and patience goes out the window. Everything requires more effort, until finally the simplest tasks seem overwhelming.

Fatigue also sabotages creativity. Judgment suffers and efficiency goes. And if unrelieved, fatigue can culminate in exhaustion and full-scale depression.

How does rest relate to these problems?

- Rest allows your body to renew itself. Waste products are removed, repairs are effected, enzymes are replenished, energy is restored.
- Rest aids in the healing of injuries, infections, and other assaults on your body, including stress and emotional traumas.
- Rest strengthens your body's immune system, helping protect you from disease.
- Proper rest can add length to your life. In a large population study of health habits a few years ago, it was found that people who regularly slept 7 to 8 hours each night had lower death rates than those who averaged either less than seven hours, or who slept longer.

How much rest do I need?

People need different kinds of rest, and a relaxing night's sleep is a good start. Newborn babies sleep from 16 to 20 hours, while young children need 10 to 12 hours. Adults vary widely in their requirements but most do best on 7 to 8 hours per night.

People also need a change of pace. During World War II, Great Britain instituted a 74-hour work week but soon found that people could not maintain the pace. After experimenting, they found that a 48-hour work week, with regular breaks, plus one day of rest each week, resulted in maximum efficiency.

Society also recognizes the need for other breaks from time to time. The long weekend is now an American institution and yearly vacations have proven their value.

What about sleep medications? Are they helpful?

During normal sleep the body passes back and forth between

periods of light and deep sleep. During light sleep dreaming occurs; this apparently provides a natural outlet for the pressures and tensions that build up during the day.

Medicated sleep, however, while producing a welcome state of unconsciousness, suppresses that dream stage. And even though people believe they have slept soundly, they may not feel as refreshed and energetic the next day.

Sleep medications may be helpful in emergencies, in other words, but they will contribute to chronic fatigue if continued over time.

Alcohol is another commonly used drug that seems to produce relaxation and aid sleep. But alcohol-induced sleep is not as restorative as normal sleep.

How can I sleep better?

- Take frequent breaks during the workday. Walk around, get a drink of water, take some deep breaths.
- Daily engage in 30 to 60 minutes of active exercise. Exercise relaxes, restores energy, helps banish depression, and combats nervous tension.
- Maintain as regular a schedule as possible for going to bed, getting up, eating, and exercising. The body flourishes on regular rhythms.
- Eat the evening meal at least four hours before bedtime. An empty, resting stomach is more conducive to quality rest.
- Try a lukewarm (not a hot) bath. It is a helpful relaxation technique.
- Count your blessings. Fill the mind with gratitude and thanksgiving.

Rest is an important part of life's rhythm. And like a dancer, if we go with our rhythms we will be in tune with ourselves.

Living the Ultimate Life

"I s this all there is?" sighs the aging baby-boomer, surrounded by his very considerable possessions. Having bought into the *grab all you can get* philosophy of the '80s, he has every material thing his heart desires. Yet, he feels curiously empty, and disappointed.

Isn't that a common human problem?

Yes, and it's getting worse. Americans are living longer, healthier lives than ever before, yet surveys show that they feel less and less satisfied.

Our hopes are continually being inflated by grandiose and unrealistic advertising, self-help gurus who promise the moon, and our childlike faith in medicine's ability to cure all our ills. As disappointments pile up, we shuffle along, looking for the missing pieces of our lives.

Are people ever really satisfied?

Early on we dream of wealth, fame, and success, of having what we want and doing as we please. But can you think of a multimillionaire athlete who isn't itching for a bigger contract? Or a wealthy celebrity who hasn't felt drawn to do yet another commercial, endorse a bigger product, or produce a new book? Where is the businessman who wouldn't jump at the next big deal or lust after another merger?

On another level, do you know a teenager who is satisfied with his/her looks? Clothes? Friends? On the face of it, humans appear to be creatures of insatiable desires.

Is this why so many people turn to drugs?

In today's fast-paced life, people often feel so pressured and stressed, so full of pain and disappointment, and so hopeless, that they become increasingly willing to gamble their health and even their lives on almost anything that promises relief, no matter how temporary. "Follow your feelings," they are urged. "If it feels good, do it." "Hurry, life is passing you by."

For every skid row bum there are scores of closet alcoholics. And for every street punk looking for a *hit,* there are many so-called respectable people numbing their pain with prescription pills.

But lasting joy doesn't come in snorts, or well-being from bottles and pills. You can't shoot up peace of mind. Gratitude and compassion aren't sold in the drugstore or on the street.

So how does one go about getting joy, peace—those good things?

The Bible says that following our "fleshly," or "natural feelings" leads to negative results like immorality, debauchery, selfish ambition, drunken orgies, fits of rage (Galatians 5:19-22, NIV).

The Bible also says that God wants better things for us, such as peace, joy, and healing. These gifts, however, come through the cultivation of our spiritual nature.

Is that kind of religious mumbo-jumbo relevant for today?

It's right on. Look at alcoholism, for instance. The medical miracles and the technological advances of the past half century have hardly touched this disease. Alcoholics Anonymous (AA) continues to offer the most consistently effective treatment with the best long-term results. AA uses a twelve-step program that involves a recognition of human helplessness and the acceptance of a Higher Power. Similar twelve-step programs, based on the philosophy of AA, are proliferating in almost every area of human need. They are bringing healing to thousands for whom medical care, drugs, counselling and other human solutions failed.

This decade is witnessing a renewed search for values, a resurgence of faith and an increasing acceptance not only of a Higher Power but of a personal, caring God.

Could this be just another fad?

This *fad* has strong roots in reality. One of the most exciting breakthroughs in recent years has been the discovery of the strong and close relationship of the physical, mental, emotional, and spiritual components of human beings.

This is a radical departure from the past because for centuries it was believed that body, mind, and spirit were separate entities that functioned independently of each other.

Now we're discovering that things like anger, fear, resentment, and distrust can actually produce effects on the body that weaken its immune system and open the door to disease. Conversely, positive emotions like love, joy, faith, and trust produce protective substances that strengthen the immune system and protect the body from disease. Harboring bitterness and hatred, nurturing negative thoughts and feelings can make us sick; cherishing positive thoughts and feelings can make us well—literally.

What does "spiritual growth" involve?

It could involve getting acquainted with your Bible, singing praise songs, and praying for the special "fruits of the Spirit" that

God wants you to possess—love, joy, peace, patience, kindness, gentleness, self-control (Galatians 5:22, 23, NIV).

We are fearfully and wonderfully made (Psalm 139:14). We don't arrive in this world, as some evolutionists claim, with only the minimal equipment needed for survival. We are each given a conscience to keep us on track; a full range of feelings and emotions to enrich our lives; and a brain that we can never use up or wear out.

Health and fitness are not enough. Neither are wealth, fame, good looks, or power. The Ultimate Lifestyle includes spiritual growth and development. It brings a contentment in which we learn that if we are not satisfied with what we have, we will never be satisfied with what we want.

Let those deep, inexplicable longings lead you to the One who can give your life hope and meaning. Spiritual growth supplies the missing pieces and fills the empty spaces. The result is a life of quality and fulfillment that will stretch into eternity.

SUMMARY

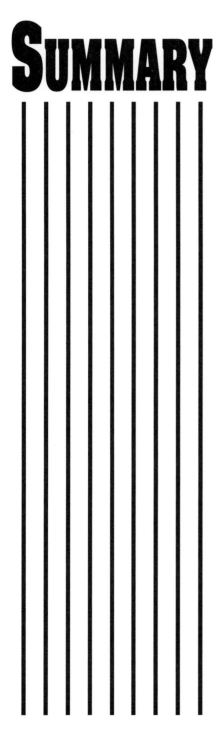

- *"Let Nutrition Be Your Medicine"*

- *Eat for Health*

- *Live for Health*

Summary

"Let Nutrition Be Your Medicine"

—*Hippocrates*

To win the battle against the epidemic of Western lifestyle diseases we must break with the lethal excesses of today's Western diet. We need a simpler, more natural way to eat.

As incredible as it might seem, there is *one* diet that not only prevents most of these killer diseases, but also helps reverse them.

Such a diet consists of a wide variety of foods eaten *as grown,* simply prepared with sparing use of fats, oils, sugars, and salt. It contains very few refined, engineered products. Animal foods, if used, are strictly limited.

Adopting this simpler, more natural dietary lifestyle brings improved health and increased energy. We can eat larger quantities of food without gaining weight, and still cut our grocery bills in half. Where, indeed, can we find a better bargain than that?

COMPARISON		
	U.S. Diet/day	**The Optimal Diet/day**
Fats & Oils	40%*	under 20%*
Sugar	35 tsp	minimal
Cholesterol	500 mg	50 mg
Salt	20 gm	5 gm
Fiber	10 gm	50 gm
Water (fluids)	minimal	8 glasses
*of total calories		

197

Eat for Health!

Basic Guidelines for a Lifetime of Good Eating

EAT LESS:

Visible fats and oils
Strictly limit fatty meats, cooking and salad oils, sauces, dressings and shortening. Use margarine and nuts very sparingly. Avoid frying; sauté instead with a little water in non-stick pans.

Sugars
Limit sugar, honey, molasses, syrups, pies, cakes, pastries, candy, cookies, soft drinks, and sugar-rich desserts—like pudding and ice cream. Save these foods for special occasions.

Foods containing cholesterol
Strictly limit meat, sausages, egg yolks, and liver. Limit dairy products, if used, to low-fat cheeses and non-fat milk products. If you eat fish and poultry, use them sparingly.

Salt
Use minimal salt during cooking. Banish the salt shaker. Strictly limit highly salted products like pickles, crackers, soy sauce, salted popcorn, nuts, chips, pretzels, and garlic salt.

Alcohol
Avoid alcohol in all forms, as well as caffeinated beverages such as coffee, colas, and black tea.

EAT MORE:

Whole grains

Freely use brown rice, millet, barley, corn, wheat, and rye. Also eat freely of whole-grain products, such as breads, pastas, shredded wheat, and tortillas.

Tubers and legumes
Freely use all kinds of white potatoes, sweet potatoes, and yams (without high-fat toppings). Enjoy peas, lentils, chick peas, and beans of every kind.

Fruits and vegetables

Eat several fresh, whole fruits every day. Limit fiber-poor fruit juices and fruits canned in syrup. Eat a variety of vegetables daily. Enjoy fresh salads with low-calorie, low-salt dressings.

Water
Drink six to eight glasses of water a day. Vary the routine with a twist of lemon and occasional herb teas.

Hearty breakfasts

Enjoy hot, multi-grain cereals, fresh fruit, and whole-wheat toast. Jumpstart your day.

Live for Health!

Basic Guidelines for a Lifetime of Healthful Living

N E W S T A R T®

NUTRITION

- Nourish your body with healthful, full-fiber, nutrient-rich foods.
- Increasingly, move toward a totally vegetarian lifestyle.
- Enhance digestion by breaking the snack habit.

EXERCISE

- Strengthen your body and increase your enjoyment of life with daily active exercise, outdoors if possible. Aim for at least 30 minutes a day. Walking is the safest exercise and one of the best.

WATER

- Come alive with an alternating hot and cold shower in the morning.
- Rinse out and refresh your insides, too, by drinking six to eight glasses of water each day.

Sunshine

- Pull back the drapes! Let the sunshine in! It will lift your spirits, brighten your day and improve your health!

Temperance

- Live a balanced life. Make time for work, play, rest, and hobbies. Nurture relationships and spiritual growth.

- Protect your body from harmful substances, such as tobacco, alcohol, caffeine, and most drugs.

Air

- Air out your house daily. Sleep in a room with good ventilation.

- Give your body a shot of oxygen by taking frequent deep breaths. Walk outdoors every day.

Rest

- Aim for seven to eight hours of sleep a night. Go to bed early enough to wake up feeling refreshed.

- Devote time to a change of pace. Attend church, go on a picnic, plant a garden, pursue a hobby, take relaxing, enjoyable vacations.

Trust

- A life of quality and fulfilment includes spiritual growth and development.

- Love, faith, trust, and hope are health-enhancing. And they bring rewards that endure.

Courtesy of the Weimar Lifestyle Program, Weimar Institute, Weimar, California 95736.

Index

I enjoyed reading
Dynamic Living.

The three most helpful chapters were:

☞ _____

_____

_____

As a result of reading this book, I have made a personal commitment to make the following changes in my lifestyle:

☞ _____

_____

_____

_____

To maintain your new lifestyle, ask for a free copy of *Lifeline* Health Letter, a 16-page magazine designed to be a pipeline of reliable health information, encouragement, and communication. Edited by Drs. Hans Diehl and Aileen Ludington, *Lifeline* is published every two months. *Lifeline* contains the latest research and practical ideas of how to improve the quality of your life and health. It's *must* reading! You may also want to enroll in the free *Way of Life* lessons.

To receive your free *Lifeline* and/or *Way of Life* lessons, simply write to

Lifestyle Medicine Institute
Dr. Hans Diehl
Loma Linda, CA 92354-0474

Dynamic Living Workbook

Hans Diehl, DrHSc, MPH
Aileen Ludington, MD
Lawson Dumbeck, MEd

E nhance your study of good health with this companion book to *Dynamic Living*. Unlike most health books, it encourages you to become personally involved through an abundance of learning exercises and activities. You will learn how to prevent and reverse heart disease, angina, diabetes (type 2), and high blood pressure, and how to cut your cholesterol and shed extra pounds while eating *more* and saving more. You will also learn how to reduce your risk of cancer, stroke, and many other lifestyle-related diseases that together account for eight of the ten leading causes of death in North America. And your medication requirements may go down!

Take charge of your health! *You* can do more for your health than any doctor, hospital, drug, or surgery. The *Dynamic Living Workbook* shows you how to do it—day by day, step by step. It shows you how to become a winner in lifestyling. Paper, 112 pages.

Ideal for individual or group study.

Available at all ABC Christian bookstores **(1-800-765-6955)** and other Christian bookstores.

Drs. Hans Diehl and Aileen Ludington are available for seminars and speaking appointments. For arrangements, please write to

Lifestyle Medicine Institute
Loma Linda, CA 92354-0474
Call 909-796-7676
or 415-692-5167

We've heard the most interesting things about you.

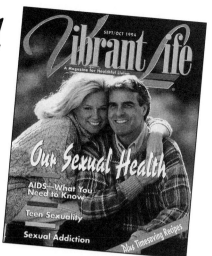

We sure have. We found out you're reducing your risk for certain cancers when you use olive oil in place of regular cooking oil. We also know which cancers you're preventing when you exercise.

Oh, we've come across lots of interesting news about you: how you can keep your defenses up against flu and colds and how much protein you *really* need.

We know you're curious about cholesterol, so we've been printing all the dependable information we could find. Do you think what you eat deserves most of the blame for a high cholesterol level? Well, you might be surprised at the truth.

We tracked down the facts you wanted on bottled waters and how much calcium you need in your diet to prevent osteoporosis.

And you should have been reading when we told how diet can slow the aging process. Really, you should be reading *Vibrant Life* all the time, because we talk a lot about you and your health. And we haven't even mentioned our articles on marriage, self-improvement, weight management, or your children's health.

Start a subscription to *Vibrant Life* today. You might find it as interesting as we find you.

For a one-year subscription (6 issues) to *Vibrant Life*, send US$8.97, Cdn$20.40, to *Vibrant Life*, P.O. Box 1119, Hagerstown, MD 21741; or call 1-800-765-6955. Add GST in Canada.

Choices

CHOICES
Quick & Healthy Cooking

MEALS YOU CAN MAKE IN 30 MINUTES OR LESS

Low in
Cholesterol, Fat
& Sodium

Cheryl Thomas Caviness
Author of Fabulous Food for Family and Friends

Create delicious, heart-healthy meals in just 30 minutes or less with Cheryl Thomas Caviness' latest cookbook. It features more than 130 recipes for creative breakfasts; portable lunches; eat-at-home lunch occasions; quick, easy dinners; and no-guilt desserts.

These meatless recipes are low in cholesterol, fat, and sodium, and each includes tips on building balanced meals; a nondairy, eggless alternative for vegan vegetarians; timesaving ideas; and complete nutritional analysis. Spiral, 144 pages. US$10.95, Cdn$15.90.

Also by Cheryl Thomas Caviness

Quick and Easy Cooking
Here's a cookbook that saves you time by showing you complete, preplanned meals for breakfast, lunch, dinner, and special occasions. Spiral, 112 pages. US$10.95, Cdn$15.90.

Fabulous Food for Family and Friends
A collection of healthy, mouthwatering menus for entertaining with style—from a picnic or barbecue to a candlelight dinner. Spiral, 128 pages. US$10.95, Cdn$15.90.

Available at all ABC Christian bookstores **(1-800-765-6955)** and other Christian bookstores. Add GST in Canada.